Student Workbook

Nutrition & Wellness for Life

Janis P. Meek, Ed.D., CFCS

Consultant and Writer
Norlina, North Carolina

Nutrition & Wellness for Life Text

by Dorothy F. West, Ph.D.

Publisher
The Goodheart-Willcox Company, Inc.
Tinley Park, Illinois
www.g-w.com

Introduction

This *Student Workbook* is designed for use with the text *Nutrition & Wellness for Life*. It is divided into chapters that correspond to the chapters in the text. By reading the text first, you will have the information you need to complete the activities in this workbook.

You will find a number of types of activities in this guide. Each chapter ends with a "Backtrack Through the Chapter" activity. This activity will help you recall the facts, interpret implications, and apply and practice chapter material. In addition, you will find activities such as crossword puzzles and fill-in-the-blank sentences. These activities will help build your vocabulary by focusing on terms introduced in the text. True-and-false and multiple-choice questions are often used to help you understand and remember text concepts. Such activities usually have specific "right" answers. You can use these activities as review guides when you study for tests and quizzes. Activities such as evaluations and comparisons will ask for opinions and ideas that cannot be judged as "right" or "wrong." These activities are designed to stimulate your thinking and help you apply text information to your daily life.

Try to complete activities without referring to the text. If necessary, you can look at the book again later to respond to any questions you could not answer. At that time, you can also compare the answers you have to the information in the book. Keep in mind that putting more thought into the activities will help you gain more knowledge from them.

Contents

Part Six   Making Informed Choices

Making Wellness a Lifestyle

Lifestyle Choices for Wellness

Activity A

Chapter 1

Name _____

Date _____ **Period** _____

Complete the left side of the chart below by listing lifestyle choices that would contribute to premature death. Complete the right side of the chart by listing choices that would contribute to optimum health. Try to include choices that relate to each of the aspects of wellness—physical health, mental health, and social health. Then answer the questions at the bottom of the page.

Premature Death ◄——————————————————————► **Optimum Health**

_____   _____
_____   _____
_____   _____
_____   _____
_____   _____
_____   _____
_____   _____
_____   _____

1. When should people adopt healthful lifestyle practices? Explain your answer. _____
   _____
   _____
   _____

2. Why do you think some people make lifestyle choices that can lead to premature death? _____
   _____
   _____
   _____

3. Besides making healthful lifestyle choices, what steps can people take to promote good health?
   _____
   _____
   _____

Words in Wellness

Use the clues provided to complete the following puzzle with key words associated with wellness.

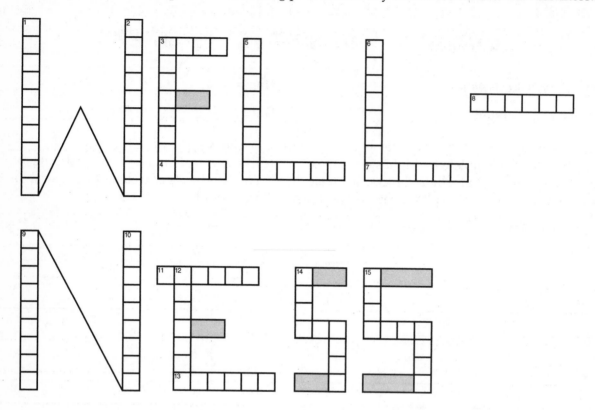

1. The average length of life of people living in the same environment is called life _____.
2. A suggested answer to a scientific question, which can be tested and verified.
3. (across) The influence people in a person's age and social group have on his or her behavior is called _____ pressure.
3. (down) The fitness of the body is _____ health.
4. A person's satisfaction with his or her looks, lifestyle, and responses to daily events is called quality of _____.
5. The state of the physical world, including the condition of water, air, and food is _____ quality.
6. A basic component of food that nourishes the body.
7. A principle that tries to explain something that happens in nature.
8. Inner agitation a person feels in response to change.
9. Death that occurs due to lifestyle behaviors that lead to a fatal accident or the formation of an avoidable disease is called _____ death.
10. The identification of a disease.
11. The way a person gets along with other people is _____ health.
12. A state of wellness characterized by peak physical, mental, and social well-being is _____ health.
13. The way a person feels about him- or herself, life, and other people is _____ health.
14. The sum of the processes by which a person takes in and uses food substances.
15. The process researchers use to find answers to their questions is called the _____ method.

Behavior-Change Contract

Name _____

Date _____ Period_____

Set a goal for improving your health this week. Use the contract below to record your goal and list specific steps you will take to reach it. Each day you complete a step, give yourself a check mark. At the end of the week, evaluate the results of your efforts by answering the questions at the bottom of the page.

Goal for Health Improvement:							
Steps	**Sun.**	**Mon.**	**Tues.**	**Wed.**	**Thurs.**	**Fri.**	**Sat.**

Evaluation

1. Are you satisfied with the results of your efforts this week? _____ Explain. _____
   _____

2. What factors helped you complete steps as planned? _____
   _____

3. What factors prevented you from completing steps? _____
   _____

4. Do you need to revise your goal or the steps you will take next week to reach it? _____ If so,
   how? _____
   _____

Evaluating Health and Nutrition Information

Activity D   **Name** _____

Chapter 1   **Date** _____ **Period**_____

Find a recent article about a health and/or nutrition research study. Attach a copy of the article to this page and answer the following questions.

1. Summarize the content and recommendations of the article.

    _____

    _____

2. In what publication or website did the article appear? _____

3. Who wrote the article? _____

    What are the author's credentials? _____

4. Who conducted the research? _____

    Describe the researchers' credentials if they are given. _____

    _____

5. Who funded the research? _____

    What do you think was the funding organization's motivation for supporting this research?

    _____

6. Describe the people who participated as study subjects. What was their gender and age range?

7. How many people did the researchers study? _____

8. For how long a period of time did the study last? _____

9. Describe how the study was set up. (For example, what traits, characteristics, or measurements were noted by researchers? How were measurements taken? Was a comparison or control group used?)

    _____

    _____

10. Does the article explain how this study compares with similar studies? If so, describe.

    _____

    _____

11. Does the article discuss further studies the researchers are doing or plan to do? If so, describe.

    _____

    _____

12. Does reading this article inspire you to make changes in your lifestyle choices? Explain why or why not.

    _____

    _____

Backtrack
Through Chapter 1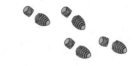

Activity E

Chapter 1

Name _____

Date _____ Period_____

Provide complete answers to the following questions and statements about making wellness a lifestyle choice.

Recall the Facts

1. What are four benefits people might notice when they begin taking steps to improve their health?
   _____

2. What are the three major components of wellness? _____
   _____

3. What is holistic medicine? _____
   _____

4. What is a risk factor? _____
   _____

5. Name four lifestyle choices that will affect a person's chances of getting a disease. _____
   _____

6. List three factors that decrease the quality of the environment. _____
   _____
   _____

7. What is one way patients sometimes interfere with the quality of their health care? _____
   _____
   _____

8. What are two reasons people develop poor health habits? _____
   _____
   _____

9. What is epidemiology? _____
   _____
   _____

10. List three main nutrition problems that are affecting the current state of wellness in the United States.
    _____
    _____

(Continued)

Interpret Implications

11. Explain in your own words the difference between mental health and social health. _____
    _____

12. Why do role expectations sometimes come into conflict? _____
    _____

13. Why is the holistic approach considered a good approach to personal health? _____
    _____

14. Explain the relationship between peer pressure and health habits. _____
    _____

15. Why is it often difficult to make changes in personal health habits? _____
    _____

16. Explain the relationship between eating habits and life expectancy. _____
    _____

Apply & Practice

17. Refer to Figure 1-1 in the text. Where would you place yourself on the wellness continuum
    today—at the center, near the "optimum health" end, or near the "premature death" end? _____
    What factors caused you to identify this point? _____
    _____

18. Give a specific example of how a teen might take a holistic approach to wellness. _____
    _____
    _____

19. If you were concerned about the mental health of a close friend, what would you do? _____
    _____
    _____

20. Describe a constructive health-related habit you have observed in the life of one of your family members.
    _____

Factors Affecting Food Choices

2

Choices in Context

Name _____

Date _____ Period _____

Read the quotes below about food choices. Identify the factor influencing each choice. Select your answers from the following list:

cultural
religious
social
emotional
historical
media
ethnic
regional
status
food biotechnology
individual preference

_____ 1. "Escargot? How can French people bear to eat snails?"

_____ 2. "Mom, let's buy that new Coco-Crunchy cereal we saw on TV."

_____ 3. "The simplest dishes always taste so much better when shared with friends at our potluck suppers!"

_____ 4. "Let's have creamed corn and sweet potatoes like the Pilgrims had for the first Thanksgiving dinner."

_____ 5. "Let's bake some brownies. That will cheer you up."

_____ 6. "We celebrate our holidays with real soul food like turnip greens and ham hocks."

_____ 7. "When I lived in the Southwest, we had tamales every Friday night."

_____ 8. "Mrs. Johnson decided to serve filet mignon because she wanted to impress her new employer."

_____ 9. "I must turn down the prime rib. Like other followers of the Hindu faith, I believe the cow is sacred."

_____ 10. "Buffalo wings are one of my favorites. I like almost anything that is hot and spicy."

_____ 11. "I'm going to try this new butter substitute just approved by the FDA. It's supposed to be better for you than butter."

How Do Friends Influence Food Choices?

Activity B

Chapter 2

Name _____

Date _____ Period _____

Interview a teen about the influence friends have on his or her food choices. Write the teen's responses to the questions below. Compile your findings with those of your classmates. Then answer the question at the bottom of the page to help you form a conclusion.

Interviewee's age _____ Interviewee's gender _____

1. Other than lunch in the school cafeteria, when was the last time you ate with friends? _____

2. How many people were in your group? _____

3. What brought your group together? _____

4. Where were you? _____

5. Would you have eaten in this location if you had been alone? Explain why or why not. _____
   _____
   _____

6. What time was it? _____

7. Would you have eaten at this time if you had been alone? Explain why or why not. _____
   _____
   _____

8. What was your mood? _____

9. What did you talk about while eating? _____

10. Did you eat a meal or a snack? _____

11. What did other people in your group eat? _____

12. What did you eat? _____

13. Would you have eaten the same food if you had been alone? Explain why or why not. _____
    _____
    _____

14. How might you have improved the nutritional value of your food choices? _____
    _____
    _____

What role do friends seem to play in influencing what, where, and when teens eat? _____
_____
_____

Food Choice Connection

Name _____

Date _____ Period _____

Match the following terms and definitions.

_____ 1. The application of a certain body of knowledge.

_____ 2. A traditional food of the African American ethnic group.

_____ 3. A belief or attitude that is important to someone.

_____ 4. The beliefs and social customs of a group of people.

_____ 5. A food prepared according to Jewish dietary laws.

_____ 6. A social custom that prohibits the use of certain edible resources as food.

_____ 7. A typical standard or pattern related to food and eating behaviors.

_____ 8. A food that has a social impact on others.

_____ 9. A food that is typical of a given racial, national, or religious culture.

_____ 10. A mainstay food in the diet.

A. culture
B. ethnic food
C. food norm
D. food taboo
E. historical food
F. kosher food
G. soul food
H. staple food
I. status food
J. technology
K. value

Quickly write any mental connections each of the following foods call to your mind. For instance, you might think a given food is fattening, feminine, or healthful. A food might make you think of a certain place, an event, or a group of people. Compare your mental connections with those of your classmates.

_____ apple

_____ burrito

_____ cheese

_____ cheeseburger

_____ chicken soup

_____ chocolate chip cookie

_____ coffee

_____ fudge

_____ milk

_____ dried plums (prunes)

_____ soda

_____ squash

Food Supply

Name _____

Date _____ Period _____

Choose a specific food item. Use various resources, such as the Internet, library references, and supermarket department managers, to investigate the supply of the item. Look for evidence of how agriculture, technology, economics, and politics have influenced the availability of the selected food. Record your findings and the resources you used in the spaces below.

Food _____

Agriculture

_____

_____

_____

_____

_____

Technology

_____

_____

_____

_____

_____

Economics

_____

_____

_____

_____

_____

_____

Politics

_____

_____

_____

_____

_____

Resources

_____

_____

Backtrack
Through Chapter 2

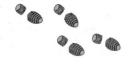

Activity E

Chapter 2

Name _____

Date _____ Period_____

Provide complete answers to the following questions and statements about factors affecting food choices.

Recall the Facts

1. What are three factors that affect people's food choices? _____

_____

2. What are four factors that helped shape your culture? _____

_____

3. What two groups of people first influenced the cuisine found in the United States today? _____

_____

4. What is an ethnic group? _____

_____

5. What are two reasons people might observe religious food customs? _____

_____

6. By watching family members, what three things might young people learn about food? _____

_____

7. What are two types of emotional responses that can be evoked by food? _____

_____

8. What kinds of problems may develop in children whose parents reward them with food? _____

_____

9. What four factors determine what foods are sold in a store? _____

_____

10. The typical diet of a region is usually based on which type of foods? _____

_____

11. What four decisions might political leaders make that would affect the food supply in a country or region?

_____

_____

12. What sources of nutrition information are most reliable? _____

_____

(Continued)

Interpret Implications

13. Why is it important to become aware of how others affect your food choices? _____
_____

14. Why must people examine the way they use food emotionally? _____
_____

15. Explain why a person's genetic makeup may cause a food to taste good or bad? _____
_____

16. How can technological advances in the areas of food production and processing help address the problem of world hunger? _____
_____

17. Explain the relationship between economics and the availability of food. _____
_____
_____

Apply & Practice

18. What is an example of a food taboo in your culture? _____
Would you consider eating this food? Explain why or why not? _____
_____
_____

19. Give an example of a status food. _____
Would you be impressed if someone served you this food? Explain why or why not. _____
_____
_____

20. What is your favorite food commercial? _____
How has this commercial influenced you? Have you been influenced to buy or try the product?
Explain why or why not. _____
_____
_____

21. What, if any, new foods or recipes have you tried as a result of watching TV cooking shows? _____
_____

22. What new food product would you like to see developed by food biotechnologists, and why?
_____

How Nutrients Become You

3

Food Breakdown

Name _____

Date _____ Period_____

Trace the steps in the process of digestion as food is broken down into simpler substances that can be used by the body. For each step, fill in the blanks with the correct word or words.

Step I: In the Mouth

1. Another word for chewing is _____.
2. Good food odors and the thought of food trigger the secretion of _____.
3. The chemical _____ _____ helps break down food starches.

Step III: In the Stomach

7. The stomach produces _____ juices to help digest food.
8. When these juices combine with chewed and swallowed food, the result is _____.
9. The gastric enzyme that begins to digest protein is _____.

Step V: In the Large Intestine

13. Another name for the large intestine is the _____.
14. The main function of the large intestine is to reabsorb _____.
15. Solid wastes that result from digestion are called _____.

Step II: In the Esophagus

4. As you swallow, food passes from the _____ to the _____.
5. The _____ prevents swallowed food from entering the windpipe.
6. The squeezing actions of muscles help move food through the esophagus. This squeezing is known as _____.

Step IV: In the Small Intestine

10. The small intestine has three parts— the_____, the _____, and the _____. Here, about 95 percent of digestion occurs.
11. The pancreas produces digestive _____ that break down fats, carbohydrates, and proteins.
12. The liver produces a digestive juice called _____, which aids digestion of fats.

What Could Be Wrong?

In each of the cases below, someone has a gastrointestinal problem. For each case, check each factor that could be affecting digestion and absorption and answer the questions.

Ruth phoned the doctor when her baby, Erica, began vomiting and developed diarrhea. The doctor asked if she had noticed any other symptoms. Then Ruth remembered the skin rash she had seen earlier when she bathed Erica. The doctor asked if Ruth had introduced any new foods into Erica's diet recently. Ruth told the doctor she had fed Erica creamed spinach for the first time that day.

1. _____ Eating habits _____ Emotions _____ Food allergy/intolerance _____ Physical activity

2. What could be wrong? _____

_____

3. What should she do? _____

_____

Charla was worried about her calculus grade. She procrastinated about studying for the next test. The night before the test, she studied until 3:00 a.m. She awoke at 7:15 a.m., grabbed a doughnut on the run, and barely made it to class by 8:00. About 45 minutes and four pages of problems later, her stomach twinges had turned into severe pains.

4. _____ Eating habits _____ Emotions _____ Food allergy/intolerance _____ Physical activity

5. What could be wrong? _____

_____

6. What should she do? _____

_____

Since he had broken his leg, Derrick hadn't been able to run or play basketball. He was also suffering from chronic indigestion. Derrick couldn't figure out what was causing it. He was eating basically the same amounts of the same foods as before.

7. _____ Eating habits _____ Emotions _____ Food allergy/intolerance _____ Physical activity

8. What could be wrong? _____

_____

9. What should he do? _____

_____

Lucas had been eating out a lot lately. Every day for a week, he had a hamburger, fries, and a milkshake for lunch. He rushed to eat so he could get back to school before sixth period. After each of these meals, Lucas felt stuffed and his stomach was upset.

10. _____ Eating habits _____ Emotions _____ Food allergy/intolerance _____ Physical activity

11. What could be wrong? _____

_____

12. What should he do? _____

_____

Digestive Disorders

Name _____

Date _____ Period_____

For each digestive disorder listed below, fill in the needed information. Describe each condition, list one or two causes of the disorder, and identify two treatments or cures available.

Diarrhea

Condition _____

Cause(s) _____

Cures _____

Constipation

Condition _____

Cause(s) _____

Cures _____

Indigestion

Condition _____

Cause(s) _____

Cures _____

Heartburn

Condition _____

Cause(s) _____

Cures _____

(Continued)

Ulcer

Condition _____

ause(s) _____

ures _____

Gallstones

Condition _____

ause(s) _____

ures _____

Diverticulosis

Condition _____

ause(s) _____

ures _____

Backtrack
Through Chapter 3

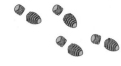

Activity D

Chapter 3

Name _____

Date _____ Period_____

Provide complete answers to the following questions and statements about how the body uses nutrients.

Recall the Facts

- -

1. Of the six types of nutrients, which are elements? _____
   Which are compounds? _____

2. Which three types of nutrients do *not* provide energy? _____

   _____

3. Explain how nutrients perform each of the following functions.
   A. Build and repair body tissues _____

   _____

   B. Regulate all body processes _____

   _____

   C. Provide energy _____

   _____

4. Give the number of calories of energy provided per gram for each of the following.
   A. Proteins _____
   B. Carbohydrates _____
   C. Fats _____
   D. Alcohol _____

5. Give one example of mechanical digestion and one example of chemical digestion. _____

   _____

6. What is an enzyme? _____

7. What role does the epiglottis play in digestion? _____

8. What is peristalsis? _____

9. How long does food usually remain in the stomach? _____

10. In which part of the body does most digestion take place? _____

11. How long does it take for food to travel from the mouth through the small intestine? _____

12. What does *metabolism* refer to? _____

   _____

(Continued)

13. What does ATP stand for and what does it do? _____

_____

14. Give two examples of emotions that can affect digestion. _____

_____

Interpret Implications

- -

15. Explain the difference between food allergy and food intolerance. _____

_____

_____

16. Explain how physical activity affects digestion and absorption. _____

_____

_____

17. Explain why laxatives are usually not needed for constipation. _____

_____

_____

18. Should ongoing or recurrent heartburn be a cause for concern? Why or why not? _____

_____

_____

Apply & Practice

- -

19. Select one personal eating habit you need to improve. Explain how this habit can affect your digestion, your body's ability to absorb nutrients, and your general wellness. _____

_____

_____

_____

_____

_____

20. List two to three strategies you use to manage emotions that can cause digestive problems. ____

_____

_____

_____

_____

_____

Nutrition Guidelines

4

Tools for Healthful Eating

Activity A

Chapter 4

Name _____

Date _____ Period_____

Read the following statements about tools for planning a healthful diet. Circle *T* if the statement is true. Circle *F* if the statement is false.

T F 1. RDAs are average daily intakes of nutrients required to meet the needs of most healthy people.

T F 2. RDA stands for *Recommended Daily Allowances*.

T F 3. RDAs are available for every known nutrient.

T F 4. The EAR of a nutrient is the recommendation estimated to meet the needs of half the people in a group.

T F 5. The UL is the amount of a nutrient you should consume every day.

T F 6. The *2010 Dietary Guidelines for Americans* focuses on maintaining calorie balance over time and consuming nutrient-dense foods.

T F 7. The *Physical Activity Guidelines for Americans* serves as the basis of most nutrition education programs in America.

T F 8. A nutrient-dense food is one that provides vitamins, minerals, and other substances that have positive health effects but supply relatively few calories.

T F 9. The *Dietary Guidelines* recommends increasing daily choices of foods that are SoFAS.

T F 10. The MyPlate system divides foods into four main food groups.

T F 11. Oils are not a food group.

T F 12. MyPlate uses volume and weight measures to describe food amounts.

T F 13. The Exchange Lists for Meal Planning system can be used to plan a healthy meal or follow a special diet.

T F 14. The Exchange Lists classify foods using the same food groups as MyPlate.

T F 15. Foods within an exchange list can be substituted for each other.

T F 16. A doctor or dietitian should determine the number of exchanges from each list needed to meet your daily requirements.

T F 17. Percent Daily Values on Nutrition Facts panels are based on a 2,000-calorie diet.

T F 18. The best times to record food intake in a food diary are holidays and special occasions.

T F 19. If you do not have a computer, you cannot do diet analysis.

Snack Inspection

Name _____

Date _____ Period_____

Compare the nutritional value of four familiar snack foods—potato chips, pretzels, tortilla chips, and a snack mix made from nuts and dried fruit. Before reading the food labels, make predictions about the nutritional value of these snacks. In the middle column of the chart below, record your predictions. Then inspect the food labels to complete the third column. Finally, write your conclusions in the space provided at the bottom of the page.

	Prediction	Inspection
1. Fewest calories		
2. Most calories		
3. Lowest sodium		
4. Lowest total fat		
5. Lowest sugar		
6. Highest saturated fat		
7. Highest trans fat		
8. Highest cholesterol		
9. Highest dietary fiber		
10. Highest protein		
11. Highest vitamin C		
12. Highest calcium		
13. Highest iron		

Conclusions:

_____

_____

_____

_____

(Continued)

Food Labels

Potato Chips

Nutrition Facts

Serving Size 1 oz. (28g/About 17 chips)
Servings Per Container 14

Amount Per Serving

Calories 160	Calories from Fat 90

	% Daily Value*
Total Fat 10g	**16%**
Saturated Fat 2g	**15%**
Trans Fat 0g	
Cholesterol 0mg	**0%**
Sodium 180mg	**8%**
Total Carbohydrate 14g	**5%**
Dietary Fiber 1g	**5%**
Sugars 0g	
Protein 2g	

Vitamin A 0%	Vitamin C 10%
Calcium 0%	Iron 0%

* Percent Daily Values are based on a 2,000 calorie diet. Your daily values may be higher or lower depending on your calorie needs:

	Calories	2,000	2,500
Total Fat	Less than	65g	80g
Sat Fat	Less than	20g	25g
Cholesterol	Less than	300mg	300mg
Sodium	Less than	2,400mg	2,400mg
Total Carbohydrate		300g	375g
Dietary Fiber		25g	30g

Calories per gram:
Fat 9   Carbohydrates 4   Protein 4

Pretzels

Nutrition Facts

Serving Size 1 oz. (28g/about 48 pretzels)
Servings Per Container 10

Amount Per Serving

Calories 110	Calories from Fat 0

	% Daily Value*
Total Fat 0g	**0%**
Saturated Fat 0g	**0%**
Trans Fat 0g	
Cholesterol 0mg	**0%**
Sodium 530mg	**22%**
Total Carbohydrate 23g	**8%**
Dietary Fiber 1g	**3%**
Sugars 1g	
Protein 3g	

Vitamin A 0%	Vitamin C 0%
Calcium 0%	Iron 8%

* Percent Daily Values are based on a 2,000 calorie diet. Your daily values may be higher or lower depending on your calorie needs:

	Calories	2,000	2,500
Total Fat	Less than	65g	80g
Sat Fat	Less than	20g	25g
Cholesterol	Less than	300mg	300mg
Sodium	Less than	2,400mg	2,400mg
Total Carbohydrate		300g	375g
Dietary Fiber		25g	30g

Calories per gram:
Fat 9   Carbohydrates 4   Protein 4

Tortilla Chips

Nutrition Facts

Serving Size 1 oz. (28g/About 6 chips)
Servings Per Container 9

Amount Per Serving

Calories 130	Calories from Fat 50

	% Daily Value*
Total Fat 6g	**9%**
Saturated Fat 1g	**9%**
Trans Fat 0g	
Cholesterol 0mg	**0%**
Sodium 80mg	**3%**
Total Carbohydrate 19g	**6%**
Dietary Fiber 1g	**5%**
Sugars 0g	
Protein 2g	

Vitamin A 0%	Vitamin C 0%
Calcium 4%	Iron 0%

* Percent Daily Values are based on a 2,000 calorie diet. Your daily values may be higher or lower depending on your calorie needs:

	Calories	2,000	2,500
Total Fat	Less than	65g	80g
Sat Fat	Less than	20g	25g
Cholesterol	Less than	300mg	300mg
Sodium	Less than	2,400mg	2,400mg
Total Carbohydrate		300g	375g
Dietary Fiber		25g	30g

Calories per gram:
Fat 9   Carbohydrates 4   Protein 4

Snack Mix

Nutrition Facts

Serving Size ¼ cup (32g)
Servings Per Container 6

Amount Per Serving

Calories 170	Calories from Fat 90

	% Daily Value*
Total Fat 11g	**17%**
Saturated Fat 3g	**15%**
Trans Fat 0g	
Polyunsaturated Fat 4g	
Monosaturated Fat 4g	
Cholesterol 0mg	**0%**
Sodium 80mg	**5%**
Potassiuum 115mg	**3%**
Total Carbohydrate 14g	**5%**
Dietary Fiber 2g	**6%**
Sugars 8g	
Protein 4g	

Vitamin A 0%	Vitamin C 2%
Calcium 2%	Iron 4%

Personal Plate

Name _____

Date _____ Period_____

For each section of the MyPlate graphic below, write in the name of the food group represented. Based on a 2,000-calorie diet, write in the recommended daily amounts for each of the five food groups. Then, list three of your favorite foods from each.

Name: _____

Amount: _____

Favorites:

1. _____

2. _____

3. _____

Name: _____

Amount: _____

Favorites:

1. _____

2. _____

3. _____

Name: _____

Amount: _____

Favorites:

1. _____

2. _____

3. _____

Name: _____

Amount: _____

Favorites:

1. _____

2. _____

3. _____

Name: _____

Amount: _____

Favorites:

1. _____

2. _____

3. _____

ChooseMyPlate.gov

Backtrack
Through Chapter 4

Activity D

Chapter 4

Name _____

Date _____ Period_____

Provide complete answers to the following questions and statements about nutrition guidelines.

Recall the Facts

1. What does each of the following tell you about a nutrient?

    A. RDA _____

    B. EAR _____

    C. AI _____

    D. UL _____

2. What groups issue the DRIs? _____

3. List the two basic themes of the *2010 Dietary Guidelines for Americans.* _____

    _____

    _____

    _____

4. What is a nutrient-dense food? _____

    _____

5. List the names of the food groups in the MyPlate system. For each group, give the daily food amounts needed for a 2,000-calorie plan. _____

    _____

    _____

    _____

6. What does the size of the food group in the MyPlate graphic represent? _____

    _____

7. For the general population, the MyPlate system creates personalized food plans based on what factors?

    _____

8. How are food amounts measured when following a MyPlate food plan? _____

    _____

9. What are the six basic lists used to classify foods in the Exchange Lists for Meal Planning?

    _____

    _____

    _____

10. What information does the Percent Daily Values on a Nutrition Facts panel give? _____

    _____

(Continued)

11. Why would a food diary be a useful tool? _____

_____

12. How can you use a computer to analyze your diet? _____

_____

13. How can you use the MyPlate system in menu planning? _____

_____

_____

Interpret Implications

14. Explain who should use DRIs and for what purposes. _____

_____

_____

_____

15. Explain why measuring food amounts is so important in learning to eat more healthfully. _____

_____

_____

_____

16. Explain why descriptions of *low* and *high nutrient density* are more useful than the terms *junk food* and *health food* in describing the quality of a food. _____

_____

_____

17. Explain why someone might want to use the Exchange Lists for Meal Planning. _____

_____

_____

_____

Apply & Practice

18. For which group or groups from the MyPlate system are you most likely to have trouble eating the recommended amounts of food? Why? _____

_____

_____

19. Identify two behaviors you could change to help you more closely follow the *Dietary Guidelines for Americans*. List four specific actions you will take to meet this goal.

_____

_____

_____

20. Use the MyPlate "Food Planner" to plan a one-day menu featuring meals and snacks that meet your nutrient needs. Write in the menu below, making sure to include all needed amounts from each food group.

_____

_____

_____

Carbohydrates: The Preferred Body Fuel 5

Carbohydrates in Action

Activity A

Chapter 5

Name _____

Date _____ Period_____

Complete the chart below by identifying what type of carbohydrate each item in the first column illustrates. Then list an example where each carbohydrate is found.

Carbohydrate	Type (mono-, di-, or polysaccharide)	Where is it found?
1. fiber		
2. fructose		
3. galactose		
4. glucose		
5. lactose		
6. maltose		
7. starch		
8. sucrose		

Plan an advertisement for a food product that is a good source of complex carbohydrates. Be creative as you answer the questions and follow the guidelines below.

What is the name of your product? _____

What is the age and gender of your intended audience? _____

Why do you think your ad will appeal to this audience? _____

_____

In what media form will your ad appear? (online, billboards, radio, TV, newspapers, magazines, other) _____

What attention-grabbing phrase or visual image will you use to open your advertisement? _____

_____

Write the main body of your ad. Be sure to explain the important functions of carbohydrates as reasons people should buy your product. _____

_____

_____

What slogan will you use at the end of your ad to help people remember your product? _____

_____

Using Carbohydrates

Name _____

Date _____ Period_____

Write the letter of the answer that best completes each statement in the space provided.

_____ 1. All carbohydrates must be in the form of _____ for cells to use them as an energy source.
A. fructose B. glucose

_____ 2. The digestive system _____ poly- and disaccharides from foods.
A. assembles B. breaks down

_____ 3. Monosaccharides travel through the _____ to the liver.
A. bloodstream B. intestines

_____ 4. The liver converts fructose and galactose into _____.
A. fat B. glucose

_____ 5. After a person eats, the amount of glucose in his or her blood _____.
A. rises B. falls

_____ 6. Insulin is released by the _____.
A. liver B. pancreas

_____ 7. Insulin helps the body _____ blood glucose to a normal level.
A. raise B. lower

_____ 8. Insulin triggers body cells to _____ glucose.
A. burn B. produce

_____ 9. If cells do not have immediate energy needs, they convert glucose to _____.
A. glycogen B. starch

_____ 10. The muscles store glycogen for use during _____.
A. muscular activity B. rest

_____ 11. The liver stores _____ of the body's glycogen.
A. one-third B. two-thirds

_____ 12. The liver can store a _____ amount of glycogen.
A. limitless B. limited

_____ 13. When someone eats more carbohydrates than the body can immediately use or store as glycogen, the liver will convert the excess into _____.
A. fat B. protein

_____ 14. Fat stores _____ be converted into glucose.
A. can B. cannot

Meeting Carbohydrate Needs

Activity C

Chapter 5

Name _____

Date _____ Period_____

Complete the chart below by listing all the foods you ate during one day from each of the indicated groups. Refer to the Exchange Lists for Meal Planning (Appendix E) in the text for a reminder of how much food equals a serving. Then write the total number of servings from each group in the space below the chart. Complete each equation to determine the approximate number of grams of carbohydrate you consumed from each group. Add the products of all the equations to determine the approximate number of grams of carbohydrate you consumed during the day. Then answer the questions at the bottom of the page.

Starch (breads, cereals and grains; starchy vegetables; crackers, snacks; and beans, peas, and lentils)
Nonstarchy Vegetables

Fruits
Milk
Sweets, Desserts, and Other Carbohydrates

	Total Servings		**Grams of Carbohydrate per Serving**		
starch	_____	×	15	=	_____
nonstarchy vegetables	_____	×	5	=	_____
fruits	_____	×	15	=	_____
milk	_____	×	12	=	_____
sweets, desserts, and other carbohydrates	_____	×	15	=	_____

Total grams of carbohydrate consumed   _____

How did your carbohydrate consumption compare to the daily recommendation of 250 to 300 grams, which is appropriate for most teens? _____

Most people in the United States need to decrease their intake of refined sugars and increase their intake of complex carbohydrates. How could you accomplish these goals? _____

_____

Chapter 5   Carbohydrates: The Preferred Body Fuel   33

"Carbs" Ahead

Activity D   **Name** _____

Chapter 5   **Date** _____ **Period** _____

Test your knowledge about issues related to carbohydrates. Fill in the blanks in the following questions. Then transfer your answers to the "billboard" and "signs" on the following page. Use the completed graphic organizer as a study aid.

1. The nutrient that provides the body's main source of energy is _____.
2. Carbohydrates composed of single sugar units are called _____.
3. The single sugar that circulates in the bloodstream is _____.
4. The single sugar that occurs in fruits and honey is _____.
5. The single sugar that is found bonded to glucose is _____.
6. Carbohydrates composed of two sugar units are called _____.
7. The sugar used in recipes or at the table is _____.
8. The sugar found in certain grains, or made of two glucose molecules that are bonded together, is _____.
9. The sugar found in milk is _____.
10. All monosaccharides and disaccharides are collectively known as _____.
11. Carbs with uncomplicated molecular structures, such as monosaccharides and disaccharides, are classified as _____ _____.
12. Carbohydrates made up of many sugar units are called _____ _____.
13. The storage form of energy in plants is _____.
14. Non-digestible carbs and binders making up cell walls in plants are _____ _____.
15. Fibers extracted from plants and prepared in a lab, such as resistant starch produced when cereals and grains are processed, are _____ _____.
16. Foods to which ingredients have been added to yield health benefits are _____ _____.
17. The sum of dietary and functional fibers is _____ _____.
18. Carbs with larger, more intricate molecular structures, such as polysaccharides, are classified as _____ _____.
19. A carbohydrate sweetener that has been separated from its original food source to be used as an additive is a _____ _____.
20. A chemical produced in the body and released into the bloodstream to regulate body processes is a _____.
21. A hormone that helps the body lower blood glucose levels is _____.
22. The body storage form of glucose is _____.
23. The feeling of fullness after eating is _____.
24. The measure of the speed at which carbs are digested, absorbed, and enter the bloodstream is _____ _____.
25. "YIELD": Do not depend on _____ to make up for poor eating habits—i.e., inadequate food sources of nutrients, including fiber.
26. "STOP" eating sticky carbs between meals to prevent _____ _____.
27. "WARNING": People with _____ _____ must regulate their sugar intake since their bodies lack, or cannot properly use, insulin to regulate blood glucose.
28. "WARNING": People with _____ need to avoid eating large amounts of sugar all at once.
29. "WARNING": People who are _____ _____ must obtain their calcium from milk alternates.

(Continued)

"Carbs" Ahead– The Preferred Body Fuel

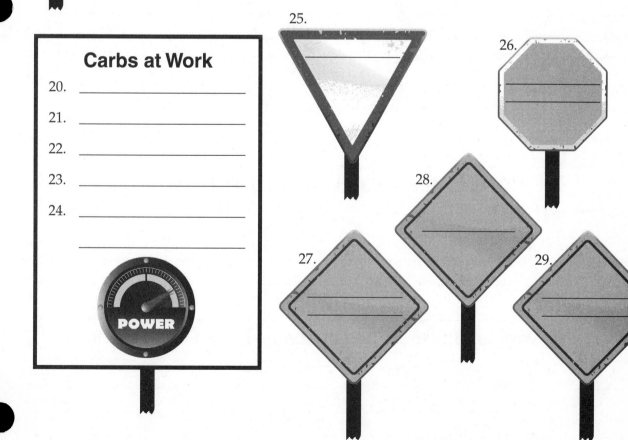

1. _____

2. _____

3. _____

4. _____

5. _____

6. _____

7. _____

8. _____

9. _____

10. _____

11. _____ _____

12. _____

13. _____

14. _____ _____

15. _____

16. _____

17. _____

18. _____

19. _____ _____

Carbs at Work

20. _____

21. _____

22. _____

23. _____

24. _____

_____

POWER

25.

26.

27.

28.

29.

Carbohydrate Headlines

Activity E

Chapter 5

Name _____

Date _____ Period_____

These tabloid headlines represent some common myths about the effects of carbohydrates in the diet. Use the space provided to write a brief rebuttal debunking each myth.

Starchy Foods Add Pounds and Inches Unlimited

_____

_____

_____

Lay Off Sweets or Lose Your Teeth!

_____

_____

_____

Kids + Sugar = HYPER!

_____

_____

_____

Sugar? Give In and Get Addicted...

_____

_____

_____

In Go the Sweets, Up Goes the Glucose—Look Out, Diabetes!

_____

_____

_____

Backtrack
Through Chapter 5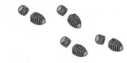

Activity F

Chapter 5

Name _____

Date _____ Period_____

Provide complete answers to the following questions and statements about carbohydrates.

Recall the Facts

1. What three components of the diet are supplied by carbohydrates? _____

   _____

2. Of what three chemical elements are carbohydrates composed? _____

3. What happens to disaccharides during digestion? _____

4. What are four foods that are high in simple carbohydrates and four foods that are high in complex carbohydrates?

   simple: _____

   complex: _____

5. What are the four key functions served by carbohydrates? _____

   _____

   _____

6. What are three diseases that may be prevented or controlled by fiber in the diet? _____

   _____

7. What are the two categories of sugars in foods? _____

   _____

8. According to the *Dietary Guidelines*, to what percent of total calories should added sugars be limited? _____

9. How many calories are provided by a gram of carbohydrates? _____

10. What are six symptoms of diabetes mellitus? _____

    _____

    _____

Interpret Implications

11. Why are carbohydrates known as the body's preferred source of energy? _____

    _____

(Continued)

12. How does carbohydrate consumption relate to the body's use of proteins? _____

_____

_____

13. How does fiber help prevent constipation, reduce the likelihood of hemorrhoids, and relieve
    diarrhea? _____

_____

_____

14. If the body converts all carbohydrates to glucose anyway, why do experts recommend eating
    more complex carbohydrates than simple sugars? _____

_____

_____

15. How can you identify foods that are high in refined sugars? _____

_____

16. Why would a dentist advise a patient to avoid snacking on sugars and starches between meals?

_____

_____

17. How might someone who is lactose intolerant meet his or her need for calcium? _____

_____

Apply & Practice

18. How many grams of fiber should you include in your diet each day? _____

19. Imagine you are giving a birthday party for a young child. Several parents express concern about
    their children coming home hyperactive from all the sweets eaten at the party. How will you
    address these concerns? _____

_____

_____

20. A friend tells you he thinks he has hypoglycemia because he gets a headache and feels shaky
    every afternoon. How would you respond? _____

_____

_____

Fats: A Concentrated Energy Source

6

Facing Fats

Activity A

Chapter 6

Name _____

Date _____ Period_____

Fill in the chart below describing types of fat, the prevalent types of fatty acids they contain, and their states at room temperature. Then answer the questions at the bottom of the page about triglycerides and other lipids.

Type of Fat	Prevalent Type of Fatty Acid	State at Room Temperature
1. beef fat		
2. corn oil		
3. olive oil		
4. soybean oil		
5. lard		
6. tropical oils		
7. peanut oil		
8. butter		
9. safflower oil		

10. Why would a manufacturer want to use hydrogenation? _____

_____

_____

11. Are trans-fatty acids better for you than saturated fatty acids? Why? _____

_____

_____

12. What is a phospholipid? _____

13. What foods contain lecithin? _____

14. Why are emulsifiers used? _____

15. Name two uses for cholesterol in the body. _____

_____

16. Which has more cholesterol—vegetable oil or animal fat? Why? _____

_____

What's My Job?

Name _____

Date _____ Period_____

Fill in the chart by listing six functions that lipids perform in the body. In the second column, give an example of each function.

Function	Example
1.	1.
2.	2.
3.	3.
4.	4.
5.	5.
6.	6.

Each "clue" below describes a part of a process involving lipids in the body. Match each clue with the appropriate term.

_____ 1. If fat is needed by the body, I break it down for immediate use. If fat is not needed right away, I convert it back to triglycerides for storage.

_____ 2. I act as an emulsifier, breaking fat into tiny droplets that can be suspended in digestive fluids.

_____ 3. I am supplied by the pancreas to break triglycerides into glycerol, fatty acids, and monoglycerides.

_____ 4. I serve as a transport line through which lipids pass on their way to the body cells.

_____ 5. With my protein and phosopholipid coat, I can carry fat but be absorbed by the lymphatic system.

_____ 6. Fat mixes with bile inside me.

_____ 7. I pick up cholesterol from around the body and transfer it to other lipoproteins, who return it to the liver.

_____ 8. I carry triglycerides and cholesterol made by the liver to the body cells so they can use them.

_____ 9. I store a limitless supply of triglycerides and send fatty acids through the bloodstream to other body cells for fuel.

_____ 10. I absorb chylomicrons before they enter the bloodstream.

_____ 11. I produce bile and cholesterol. I also process returned cholesterol as a waste product for removal from the body.

_____ 12. I carry cholesterol (not triglycerides) through the bloodstream to the body.

_____ 13. I am one of four special combinations of fat and protein that help transport fats in the body.

A. bile

B. bloodstream

C. body cell

D. chylomicrons

E. enzymes

F. fat cells

G. HDL

H. large intestine

I. LDL

J. lipoproteins

K. liver

L. lymphatic system

M. small intestine

N. VLDL

Recognize the Risks

Name _____

Date _____ Period_____

In each of the following pairs, place an R in the blank beside the description of the person with the greater risk for coronary heart disease. Then answer the questions at the bottom of the page.

1. _____25-year-old   _____60-year-old

2. _____male   _____female

3. _____African American   _____Asian American

4. _____second cousin had a heart attack   _____father has high blood pressure

5. _____overweight   _____underweight

6. _____chain-smoker   _____nonsmoker

7. _____low-fat diet   _____high-fat diet

8. _____active lifestyle   _____sedentary lifestyle

9. _____irritable, impatient personality   _____mild personality traits

10. _____low-stress work   _____normal-stress work

11. _____normal blood pressure   _____high blood pressure

12. _____diabetic   _____nondiabetic

13. _____high serum cholesterol   _____low serum cholesterol

14. Of the risk factors listed in the chapter, which are uncontrollable? _____

_____

_____

_____

15. Which are controllable? _____

_____

_____

_____

16. For each risk factor that is controllable, explain what a person could do to lower his or her risk.

_____

_____

_____

_____

_____

_____

_____

Heart of the Matter

Name _____

Date _____ Period_____

For each row in the puzzle, write in the correct term from the chapter. Use the numbered clues to help you.

1. A substance, such as a phospholipid, that can mix with water and fat.
2. The death of heart tissue caused by blockage of an artery carrying nutrients and oxygen to that tissue.
3. A fatty acid that forms when oils are partially hydrogenated.
4. A(n) _____ fatty acid has only one double bond between carbon atoms in a carbon atom chain.
5. The body stores lipids in _____ tissue.
6. A fat that has spoiled, giving it an unpleasant smell and taste.
7. Lipids with a phosphorus-containing compound in their chemical structure. They can combine with both fat and water to form emulsions.
8. _____ disease is the name for disease of the heart and blood vessels.
9. A phospholipid made by the liver and found in many foods.
10. _____-3 fatty acids are a type of polyunsaturated fatty acids found in fish oils. They have been shown to have a positive effect on heart health.
11. The body cannot make this type of fatty acid, but it is needed for normal growth and development, so it must be supplied by the diet.
12. A(n) _____ fatty acid has at least one double bond between two carbon atoms in each molecule and, therefore, is missing at least two hydrogen atoms.
13. Fat droplets that are coated by proteins so they can be transported in the bloodstream.
14. A(n) _____ fatty acid has no double bonds in its chemical structure and, therefore, carries a full load of hydrogen atoms.
15. An organic compound that is made up of a chain of carbon atoms to which hydrogen atoms are attached. It has an acid group at one end.
16. A white, waxy lipid made by the body that is part of every cell. It is also found in foods of animal origin.
17. A group of compounds that includes triglycerides, phospholipids, and sterols.
18. A(n) _____ lipoprotein picks up cholesterol from around the body and transfers it to other lipoproteins for transport back to the liver for removal from the body.
19. A(n) _____ fatty acid that has two or more double bonds between carbon atoms in a carbon atom chain.
20. The process of breaking the double carbon bonds in unsaturated fatty acids and adding hydrogen to make the fatty acid more saturated.
21. A(n) _____-density lipoprotein carries triglycerides and cholesterol made by the liver through the bloodstream to the body.
22. The major type of fat found in foods and in the body. It consists of three fatty acids attached to a glycerol molecule.
23. Abnormally high blood pressure; an excess force on the walls of the arteries as blood is pumped from the heart.
24. A condition of hardened and narrowed arteries caused by plaque deposits.
25. A medical test that measures the amounts of cholesterol, triglycerides, HDL, and LDL in the blood is a(n) _____ profile.
26. A buildup of fatty compounds made up largely of cholesterol that form on the inside walls of arteries.
27. The death of brain tissue caused by blockage of an artery carrying nutrients and oxygen to that tissue.
28. A cluster of triglycerides that is thinly coated with cholesterol, phospholipids, and proteins. It is absorbed into the lymphatic system and eventually moved into the bloodstream.
29. An ingredient used in food products to replace some or all the fat typically found in those products.

(Continued)

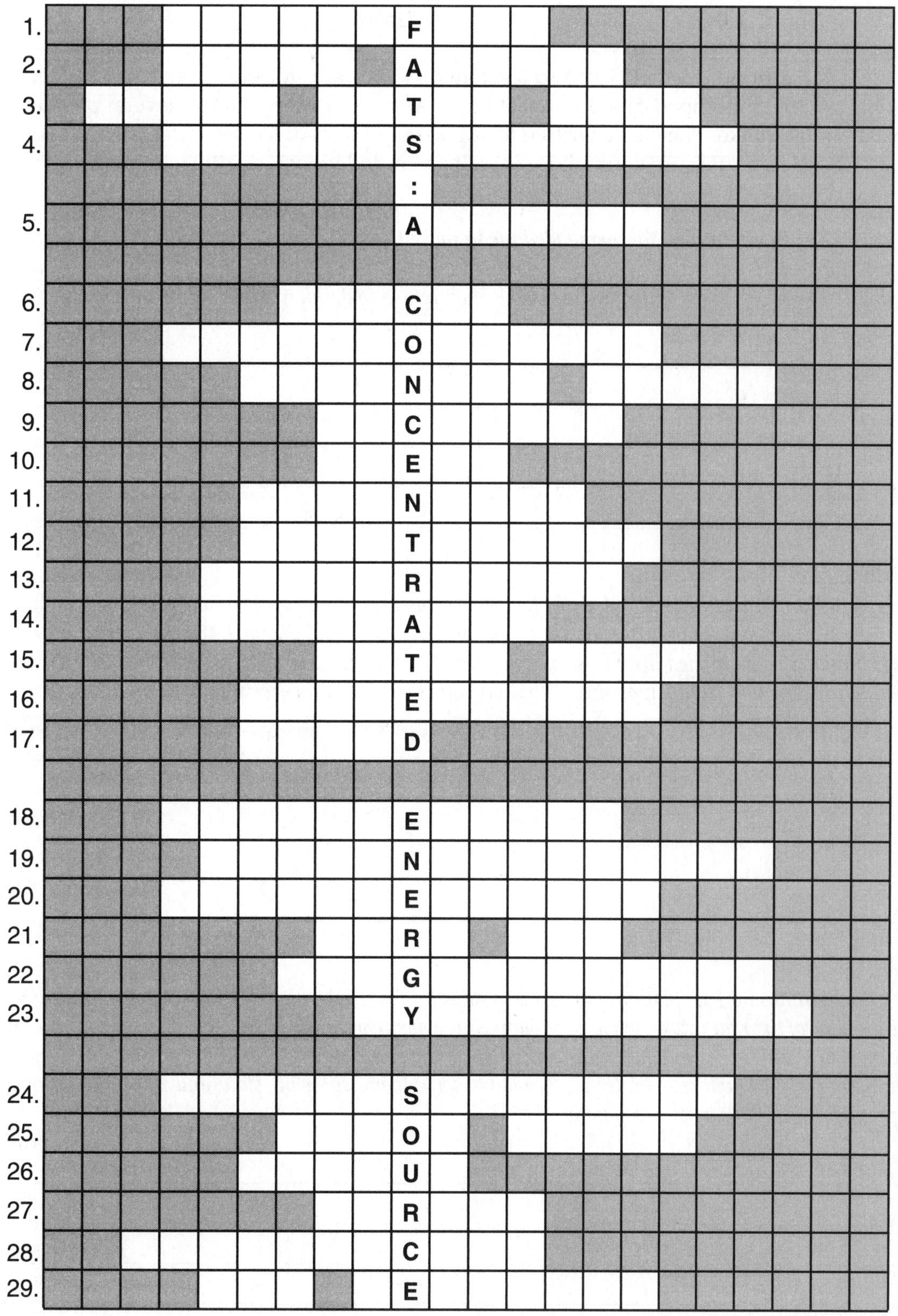
1. F
2. A
3. T
4. S
:
5. A
6. C
7. O
8. N
9. C
10. E
11. N
12. T
13. R
14. A
15. T
16. E
17. D
18. E
19. N
20. E
21. R
22. G
23. Y
24. S
25. O
26. U
27. R
28. C
29. E

Letters from Low-Fat Lane

Activity E

Chapter 6

Name _____

Date _____ Period_____

Pretend you are a community dietitian. You teach nutrition classes for groups in your community. Your last class was at a neighborhood called Low-Fat Lane. After your presentation, several people still had questions about fat intake. They have written to you asking your advice. Read each letter and respond to the person's concerns. Be sure your advice is well grounded in factual information from the text.

Dear Dietitian:

I enjoyed your presentation. You persuaded me to make the switch from whole milk to fat-free milk in my household. Unfortunately, I haven't been very successful. My husband and sons are giving me a hard time over it. They just don't like the taste of the fat-free milk! They refuse to drink it. How can I convince them?

Minus the Milkfat Mom

_____

_____

_____

_____

Dear Dietitian:

My friend Flora Foster is paranoid about fat. She seems to be going overboard in her search for a fat-free life. When she took her son, Freddy, for his six-week checkup, she asked the pediatrician if he could recommend a fat-free formula. She is worried little Freddy will grow up to be obese like his grandfather. She wants to start right away to prevent that from happening. What do you think about fat-free infant formula?

Flustered over Flora

_____

_____

_____

_____

_____

Dear Dietitian:

My wife, Franny, and I are planning to host a cookout for the neighborhood this weekend. Our new neighbors are very conscious of their fat intake, so we have planned the menu accordingly. We aren't having steaks, because they have marbling and fat around the edges. Instead, we're serving hot dogs. They offer smaller portions and less visible fat. Since our meal will be so healthful, we plan to serve them with chili, slaw, and all the trimmings! Thanks for your presentation. We're on our way now!

Heart-Healthy Hosts

_____

_____

_____

_____

_____

(Continued)

Dear Dietitian:

    My cousin Faith is working hard to lose 50 pounds as her doctor recommended. She has cut down her fat intake and kept a daily food diary for the last three months. She seems to be making some progress. When I saw Faith the other day, she said she has lost eight pounds. Her only complaint was that it seemed to be taking forever. I didn't know what to say to her. What do you think? Is there anything I can do to help her?

Concerned Clara

_____

_____

_____

_____

_____

Dear Dietitian:

    My husband, Fritz, took me out to dinner last night. We had grilled chicken, fat-free dressing on the salad, and baked potatoes. We topped it off with the dessert specialty of the house, "Death by Chocolate." We figured it was okay to splurge, since we had eaten such a smart meal! Were we right?

Wondering Wanda

_____

_____

_____

_____

_____

Dear Dietitian:

    At your presentation, you briefly mentioned fat replacers. I want to know more about them. Are they safe? Do products that use them taste the same as regular products? Are they lower in calories? Where can I find them?

Inquisitive Irene

_____

_____

_____

_____

_____

Dear Dietitian:

    I am trying to eat more healthfully. I have been eating fish instead of higher-fat meats. I found that if I fry the fish in oil and serve it with French fries, it tastes pretty good. When I'm really on top of it, I add a small vegetable salad with lots of salad dressing and cornbread with lots of butter. I'm so glad you advised me to eat more fish. Thanks!

Crazy for Catfish

_____

_____

_____

_____

_____

Backtrack
Through Chapter 6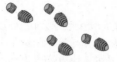

Activity F

Chapter 6

Name _____

Date _____ Period _____

Provide complete answers to the following questions and statements about fats.

Recall the Facts

1. What is the composition of triglycerides? _____
   _____

2. Which fats tend to be higher in saturated fatty acids—those from animals or those from plants?

3. What are the two main reasons for hydrogenating oils? _____
   _____

4. Why is lecithin important in the making of homemade mayonnaise? _____
   _____

5. Why are lecithin and cholesterol not essential in the diet? _____
   _____

6. Give three examples of sterols. _____

7. How do lipids reach body tissues? _____
   _____

8. What is the leading cause of death in the United States? _____

9. Why do young females tend to have less risk for heart disease than young males? _____
   _____

10. List seven controllable factors that affect heart health. _____
    _____
    _____
    _____

11. Name four ways exercise can have a positive effect on heart health. _____
    _____
    _____

12. What is the relationship between fat in the diet and risk for cancer? _____
    _____

(Continued)

● Interpret Implications

- -

13. Why is the word *lipid* considered broader than the word *fat*? _____

_____

_____

14. Explain the difference between LDL and HDL. _____

_____

_____

_____

_____

15. Explain how plaque buildup in the arteries causes high blood pressure. _____

_____

_____

_____

_____

16. Explain why some cholesterol is termed "good" and some is termed "bad." _____

_____

_____

_____

_____

17. An article reported that native Alaskans who consumed a lot of fish oil had a low rate of CHD. Would it then be wise to conclude taking fish oil pills would reduce the risk of heart attack? Why?

_____

_____

_____

_____

Apply & Practice

- -

18. What was the most startling fact you learned about fats from reading the chapter? How will you use this information to help you eat more healthfully? _____

_____

_____

_____

(Continued)

19. Your friend has an overweight mother and a father with high blood pressure. She has gone on a totally fat-free diet because she wants to stay slim and healthy. What advice would you offer her?

_____

_____

_____

20. List four ways you can modify your diet to limit fats and cholesterol. _____

_____

_____

_____

Proteins: The Body's Building Blocks   7

Building Blocks of Protein

Name _____

Date _____ Period_____

Choose the best response to complete each multiple choice statement. Write the letter for each answer in the block below containing the same number as the statement. Your answers will reveal an essential component of proteins.

1	2	3	4	5
6	7	8	9	10

_____ 1. Protein differs from carbohydrates and fats because of the _____ it contains.
    A. nitrogen   B. oxygen   C. hydrogen   D. carbon

_____ 2. Protein makes up about _____ percent of your body.
    L. 12 to 15   M. 18 to 20   N. 20 to 25   O. 30 to 40

_____ 3. When proteins change shape and take on new characteristics, _____ has occurred.
    G. balance   H. completion   I. denaturation   J. coagulation

_____ 4. To say the body can synthesize a compound means that it can _____ it.
    L. destroy   M. digest   N. make   O. complement

_____ 5. There are _____ indispensable amino acids.
    L. 20   M. 19   N. 11   O. 9

_____ 6. Proteins that defend the body against infection and disease are _____.
    A. antibodies   B. buffers   C. enzymes   D. hormones

_____ 7. The liver converts nitrogen waste from proteins into _____.
    A. enzymes   B. lipoproteins C. urea   D. urine

_____ 8. Plants that can capture nitrogen from the air and transfer it to their protein-rich seeds are _____.
    G. grains   H. hummus   I. legumes   J. tofu

_____ 9. Complete proteins come from _____ sources.
    A. plant and animal B. only plant   C. only mineral   D. only animal

_____ 10. Two incomplete proteins that together provide all the indispensable amino acids are said to be _____.
    Q. complete   R. animal   S. complementary T. valuable

A Billboard for Proteins

Activity B   **Name** _____

Chapter 7   **Date** _____ **Period**_____

In the space provided below, list the six basic functions of protein in the body. Then design a billboard to advertise one of the functions. Choose a function and write a summary of the message of your design. Use the box at the bottom of the page to illustrate your billboard. Be sure to use an attention-getting slogan, logo, and layout.

Functions of Protein

1. _____   4. _____

2. _____   5. _____

3. _____   6. _____

Summary of Message

_____

_____

_____

Animal vs. Plant Proteins

Name _____

Date _____ Period_____

Complete the following chart to contrast plant and animal proteins. Supply the information called for in each row of the chart. Then answer the question at the bottom of the page.

	Animal Sources of Protein	Plant Sources of Protein
Examples		
Protein Quality		
Advantages		
Disadvantages		

Do you choose more protein from plant sources or animal sources? Explain your response.

_____

_____

_____

Complementary Proteins—A "Good Match"

Name _____

Date _____ Period_____

For each of the following recipes, circle the ingredients that are complementary sources of protein. Use a recipe book to find a third example of a recipe containing complementary proteins. Write the name of the recipe on the tab of the third recipe card below. List the ingredients for the recipe on the lines of the card. Then circle the complementary sources of protein contained in the recipe.

Vegetarian Chili Mac

3	cups canned tomatoes		1	tablespoon oil
¾	cup uncooked whole-grain macaroni		2	teaspoons chili powder
¾	cup chopped onion		1	teaspoon dried basil
2	cloves garlic, crushed		3	cups canned kidney beans
¼	cup chopped green pepper			

Stir-Fried Vegetables and Tofu

1	cup orange-ginger sauce		1	medium red bell pepper
2	tablespoons peanut oil		½	pound mushrooms
1	medium onion		1	cup bean sprouts
2	carrots		1½	cups diced firm tofu
2	ribs celery		6	cups cooked brown rice
2	cups broccoli florets			

_____
_____
_____
_____
_____
_____
_____

Protein Balance

Name _____

Date _____ Period_____

Decide which of the following statements about protein needs are true and which are false. Write the numbers of statements that are true inside the blocks on the left end of the scale. Write the numbers of those that are false on the right end. If you have identified the statements correctly, you will have the same number on each end, thus preserving the "protein balance."

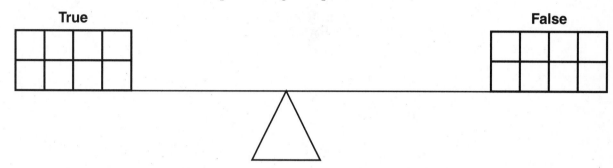

1. The human body can store excess amino acids as a protein source.

2. The most important factor in determining how much protein a person needs is his or her activity level.

3. Most people in the United States eat more protein than they need.

4. Children need proportionally more protein than adults.

5. Extra protein is needed to support the growth of unborn babies in pregnant women and the production of milk in breast-feeding mothers.

6. In general, females require more protein than men of the same age and size.

7. A large, tall person needs more protein than a small, short person.

8. Sick people require extra protein to build antibodies.

9. The RDAs for protein include a margin of safety.

10. For people between the ages of 4 and 18, the DRI for protein is 20 percent of calories.

11. The Nutrition Facts panel on food products can help people estimate how much protein they consume each day.

12. People who exercise occasionally need extra protein to build muscle and supply energy.

13. Athletes should consume more calories from protein than from carbohydrates.

14. The grains and vegetable groups of the MyPlate system are the primary food sources of protein.

15. One-fourth cup of cooked legumes counts as a one ounce-equivalent of protein.

16. People can avoid health risks by choosing protein sources that are high in saturated fats.

Not Too Little—Not Too Much

Name _____

Date _____ Period_____

Use the clues provided to identify conditions brought on by too little or too much protein in the diet. Write one letter in each space; do not leave blank spaces between words. Note the first four answers are in the "plus zone," reflecting too much protein intake. The last four answers are in the "minus zone," reflecting too little protein intake.

"Plus Zone"

1. __ __ __ __ __ __

2. __ __ __ __ __ __ __ __ __

3. __ __ __ __ __ __ a n d __ __ __ __ __ __ __ __

4. __

Protein•Protein•Protein•Protein•Protein•Protein•Protein•Protein•Protein•Protein

5. __ __ __ __ __ __ __ - __ __ __ __ __ __ __ __ __ __ __ __ __ __ __ __ __

6. __

7. __ __ __ __ __ __ __ __ __ __ __ __

8. __ __ __ __ __ __ __ __ __

"Minus Zone"

1. Since many high-protein foods are also high-fat foods, the result of a high-protein diet may be excess _____ _____.

2. When a person consumes a diet high in protein from animal sources, he or she may develop _____ _____ in the bones.

3. A high-protein diet creates extra work for the _____ and _____, the organs responsible for handling nitrogen waste.

4. A person who takes in more protein than he or she excretes is in _____ _____ _____.

5. A lack of calories and proteins in the diet causes a condition called _____-_____ _____.

6. A person who loses more nitrogen than he or she consumes is in _____ _____ _____.

7. When mothers in poor countries wean older children to begin breast-feeding newborns, the older children may develop _____.

8. The muscles and tissues of people suffering from starvation begin to waste away due to a PEM disease called _____.

Backtrack
Through Chapter 7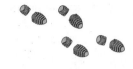

Activity G

Chapter 7

Name _____

Date _____ Period_____

Provide complete answers to the following questions and statements about proteins.

Recall the Facts

- -

1. Of what four elements are proteins composed? _____

   _____

2. What are four factors or substances that can denature proteins? _____

   _____

3. How many amino acids are needed for good health? _____ How many of the amino acids are indispensable? _____ How many are dispensable? _____

4. What are six functions of proteins in the body? _____

   _____

   _____

5. What are three important compounds the body makes from proteins? _____

   _____

6. What are three vital substances that are carried by proteins in the bloodstream? _____

   _____

7. What are four factors that influence protein food choices? _____

   _____

   _____

8. Name six types of legumes. _____

   _____

9. What are three positive factors associated with plant sources of protein in terms of heart health and cancer risk reduction? _____

   _____

   _____

10. What four factors determine the amount of protein you need? _____

   _____

   _____

(Continued)

Copyright by Goodheart-Willcox Co., Inc.

Chapter 7 Proteins: The Body's Building Blocks   55

11. What groups of the MyPlate system are the primary food sources of protein? _____

_____

12. What population group is often affected by kwashiorkor? _____

_____

Interpret Implications

- -

13. Explain why adults need dietary protein even though they have reached their growth potential.

_____

14. Explain why proteins are not considered the preferred source of body energy. _____

_____

_____

15. Explain the difference between complete proteins and incomplete proteins. _____

_____

_____

16. What factors impact an athlete's protein needs during exercise? _____

_____

17. Why is nitrogen balance used to evaluate a person's protein status? _____

_____

Apply & Practice

- -

18. What protein source would you choose to complement whole-grain bread when serving lunch to a vegetarian friend? Explain your choice. _____

_____

_____

19. What is your RDA for protein? _____

20. Suppose your friend is a body builder. He tells you he has been following a high-protein diet and consuming amino acid supplements to help increase his muscle mass. Describe and explain your response. _____

_____

_____

_____

Vitamin Analogies

Activity A

Chapter 8

Name _____

Date _____ Period_____

For each analogy given, underline the term from the parentheses that best completes the analogy. (An *analogy* is a comparison between two sets of concepts. For example, "vitamins : body processes :: thermostat : room temperature" is read "vitamins are to body processes as a thermostat is to room temperature." This analogy means vitamins regulate body processes just as thermostats regulate room temperatures.)

1. provitamin : vitamin :: beta-carotene : (thiamin, vitamin A, vitamin C, vitamin D)

2. fat-soluble : vitamins A, D, E and K :: water-soluble : (thiamin and riboflavin, folate and niacin, B vitamins and vitamin C, biotin and thiamin)

3. food poisoning : foodborne bacteria :: toxicity : (large doses of supplements, vitamin deficiencies, undernourishment, malabsorption)

4. epithelial cells : human body :: (windows, siding, flooring, plumbing) : house

5. riboflavin : inflamed tongue :: vitamin A : (crossed eyes, night blindness, cataracts, glaucoma)

6. enriched : breads :: fortified : (fruits, vegetables, dairy products, meats)

7. children : adults :: rickets : (osteomalacia, osteoporosis, skin cancer, heart disease)

8. (vitamin A, vitamin C, vitamin D, vitamin K) : osteomalacia :: thiamin : beriberi

9. antioxidant : protection from oxygen exposure :: free radical : (tissue growth, tissue damage, tissue exposure, tissue transformation)

10. folate deficiency : neural tube :: vitamin E deficiency : (plasma, white blood cells, red blood cells, iron)

11. incineration : burning :: coagulation : (bleeding, hemorrhaging, clotting, bandaging)

12. car : wheels :: inactive enzyme : (provitamins, coenzymes, enzymes, complex)

13. alcoholic : thiamin :: smoker : (vitamin A, vitamin C, vitamin D, vitamin K)

14. scurvy : vitamin C :: beriberi : (thiamin, riboflavin, niacin, biotin)

15. niacin flush : toxicity :: (pellagra, pernicious anemia, rickets, erythrocyte hemolysis) : deficiency

16. cement : bricks :: (plasma, antioxidant, collagen, choline) : cells

17. pellagra : flaky skin :: pernicious anemia : (vitality, diarrhea, skin tingling, rash)

18. probiotics : "good" microorganisms :: (coagulants, deficiencies, flavonoids, provitamins) : phytochemicals

Vitamin Sources and Functions

Name _____

Date _____ Period_____

Use a food composition table or other reliable source to complete the chart below. For each vitamin, list foods that are good sources. Then list functions of the vitamin in the body, the classification (whether the vitamin is fat-soluble or water-soluble), and the RDA or AI recommendation for someone of your age and gender.

Vitamin	Food Sources	Functions	Classification	RDA or AI
1. biotin				
2. folate				
3. niacin				
4. pantothenic acid				
5. riboflavin				
6. thiamin				
7. vitamin A				
8. vitamin B_6				
9. vitamin B_{12}				
10. vitamin C				
11. vitamin D				
12. vitamin E				
13. vitamin K				

Cause and Effect

Name _____

Date _____ Period_____

Fill in the missing information to complete the chart below. In some cases, you will need to provide the cause of the problem that is given. In other cases, you will list the effect of the deficiency or excess given.

Cause	Effect
1.	1. Night blindness
2.	2. Beriberi
3. Riboflavin deficiency	3.
4.	4. Rickets
5. Vitamin E deficiency in premature babies	5.
6.	6. Nausea; loss of appetite; dry, scaly skin; abnormal heart rhythms
7. Excess vitamin A	7.
8. Large doses of vitamin B$_6$	8.
9.	9. Jaundice
10. Folate deficiency	10.
11.	11. Pellagra
12. Inability to absorb vitamin B$_{12}$	12.
13. Vitamin D excess	13.
14.	14. Scurvy
15. Toxic levels of niacin	15.
16. Megadoses of vitamin C	16.

Foods vs. Supplements

Name _____

Date _____ Period_____

Use the space provided to compare and contrast the benefits of getting vitamins from supplements with those of getting vitamins from food sources.

Benefits of Vitamin Supplements

_____

_____

_____

_____

_____

_____

_____

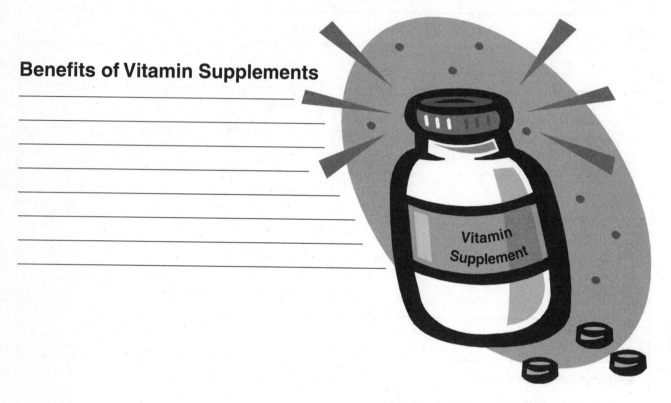

Benefits of Vitamins from Foods

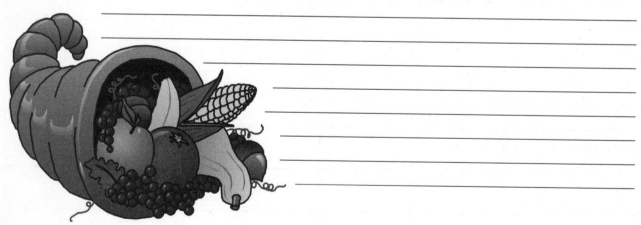

_____

_____

_____

_____

_____

_____

Viva Las Vitamins!

Name _____

Date _____ Period_____

"Long live the vitamins!" Except in special circumstances, a balanced diet supplies all the vitamins needed by the body. Unfortunately, many vitamins are needlessly lost due to poorly chosen methods for food selection, preparation, and storage. Use the boxes provided to design mini-posters about preservation of vitamins in foods.

Food Selection

(Continued)

Food Preparation

Food Storage

Backtrack
Through Chapter 8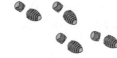

Activity F

Chapter 8

Name _____

Date _____ Period_____

Provide complete answers to the following questions and statements about vitamins.

Recall the Facts

- -

1. How many calories per gram do vitamins provide? _____

2. Why does the body need vitamins? _____

3. What makes vitamins organic compounds? _____

   _____

4. How long does it usually take for a vitamin deficiency to produce first symptoms? _____

5. Name three stages in the life cycle during which the body has a greater than usual need for vitamins.

   _____

6. What is toxicity and how does it relate to vitamin consumption? _____

   _____

7. What is a unit of measurement for vitamin A other than the microgram? _____

8. What nutrient can be produced by the body through exposure to sunshine? _____

9. Intestinal bacteria can produce what useful vitamin? _____

10. Name the eight B vitamins. _____

    _____

11. What is a coenzyme and what does it do? _____

    _____

12. What causes scurvy? _____

13. What are the benefits of phytochemicals, and how can you realize these benefits? _____

    _____

Interpret Implications

- -

14. Explain the relationship between antioxidants and free radicals. What vitamins are antioxidants?

    _____

    _____

(Continued)

15. A dietitian works for a program for recovering alcoholics. What vitamin deficiency do you think the dietitian is most likely to encounter among her clients and why? _____

_____

_____

16. Why do health experts recommend females increase their daily intake of folate between puberty and menopause? _____

_____

_____

17. In most cases, the best way to supply the body with needed vitamins is from food items or from vitamin supplements. Explain.

_____

_____

18. List four ways foods can lose vitamins. For each way listed, suggest a way this vitamin loss can be prevented.

_____

_____

_____

_____

Apply & Practice

19. Write five personal goals you could set to help you meet all your vitamin needs.

_____

_____

_____

_____

_____

20. A flyer is being distributed outside a health foods store. The flyer promotes the sale of a vitamin E product by making the following claims:

Vitamin E...An Answer for Every Ailment...

$\mathcal{E}+$
- *Maintains youthful vim, vigor, and vitality*
- *Maintains a healthy immune system*
- *Sustains peak performance*
- *Prevents tissue damage*
- *Protects blood cells*

Which claims are valid?

_____

Which are invalid?

_____

Minerals: Regulators of Body Functions 9

Mineral Match

Activity A

Chapter 9

Name _____

Date _____ Period_____

Match the following terms and identifying phrases.

_____ 1. An inorganic element needed in small amounts to perform various functions in the body.

_____ 2. Mineral required in the diet in an amount of 100 or more milligrams per day.

_____ 3. Mineral required in the diet in an amount of less than 100 milligrams per day.

_____ 4. A condition that results when bones become porous and fragile due to a loss of calcium.

_____ 5. The time in a woman's life when menstruation ends due to a decrease in production of the hormone estrogen.

_____ 6. An abnormal cessation of menstrual periods.

_____ 7. The movement of water across cell membranes to equalize the concentrations of mineral particles on each side of the membrane.

_____ 8. A compound that has a pH lower than 7.

_____ 9. A term used to express the measure of a substance's acidity or alkalinity.

_____ 10. An iron-containing protein that helps red blood cells carry oxygen from the lungs to cells throughout the body and carbon dioxide from body tissues back to the lungs for excretion.

_____ 11. A condition in which the number of red blood cells decline, causing the blood to have a decreased ability to carry oxygen to body tissues.

_____ 12. A substance that acts with enzymes to increase enzyme activity.

_____ 13. A hormone produced by the thyroid gland that helps control metabolism.

_____ 14. An enlargement of the thyroid gland.

_____ 15. Severe mental retardation and dwarfed physical features of a child caused by the mother's iodine deficiency during pregnancy.

_____ 16. A spotty discoloration of teeth caused by high fluoride intake.

A. acid
B. amenorrhea
C. base
D. cofactor
E. cretinism
F. fluorosis
G. goiter
H. hemoglobin
I. iron-deficiency anemia
J. macromineral
K. menopause
L. micromineral
M. mineral
N. myoglobin
O. osmosis
P. osteoporosis
Q. pH
R. thyroxine

Go to the Source

Name _____

Date _____ Period_____

Complete the following chart by listing functions and food sources of each of the listed minerals. Then answer the questions at the bottom of the page.

Minerals	Functions	Sources
Calcium		
Phosphorus		
Magnesium		
Sulfur		
Sodium		
Potassium		
Chloride		
Iron		
Zinc		
Iodine		
Fluoride		
Selenium		
Copper		
Chromium		
Manganese		
Molybdenum		

Do you eat food sources of each of the above minerals every day? _____

If not, which minerals may be lacking in your diet?_____

_____

Mineral Mysteries

Choose the best response to complete each statement about mineral deficiencies and excesses. Write the letter in the space provided.

_____ 1. A gradual loss of bone density can result from a deficiency of _____.

A. calcium   B. magnesium   C. phosphorus   D. sulfur

_____ 2. A great excess of _____ in the diet can cause fluorosis.

A. chloride   B. fluoride   C. potassium   D. sodium

_____ 3. A deficiency of _____ can result in anemia.

A. copper   B. fluoride   C. iodine   D. zinc

_____ 4. Excessive amounts of _____ can cause liver damage and is a leading cause of accidental poisoning among children in the U.S.

A. copper   B. chromium   C. iron   D. selenium

_____ 5. For people who are sensitive to this mineral, excess _____ can provoke hypertension.

A. calcium   B. manganese   C. molybdenum   D. sodium

_____ 6. Goiter may be the result of a(n) _____ deficiency.

A. magnesium   B. iodine   C. iron   D. phosphorus

_____ 7. Heart malfunction, along with muscle cramps, constipation, loss of appetite, and confusion, can be symptoms of a _____ deficiency.

A. calcium   B. potassium   C. iodine   D. sulfur

_____ 8. Impaired glucose metabolism may be caused by a deficiency of _____.

A. calcium   B. chloride   C. chromium   D. copper

_____ 9. Nausea, hair loss, and nerve damage are symptoms associated with an excess of _____.

A. selenium   B. sodium   C. sulfur   D. zinc

_____ 10. Poor calcium absorption can be caused by excess _____ in the diet.

A. fluoride   B. iodine   C. phosphorus   D. potassium

_____ 11. The most common type of anemia is caused by a deficiency of _____.

A. copper   B. iodine   C. iron   D. selenium

_____ 12. Weakness, heart irregularities, disorientation, and seizures may result from a low intake of _____.

A. calcium   B. magnesium   C. manganese   D. molybdenum

Minerals, More or Less

Name _____

Date _____ Period_____

Fill in the blank in each statement with either the word *more* or the word *less*.

1. Studying about mineral sources and functions can help people make _____ healthful decisions about foods.

2. Crops grown in soil that lacks minerals will contain _____ minerals than crops grown in mineral-rich soil.

3. _____ minerals are located in the outer layers of grain than in the inner parts.

4. _____ minerals are found near the peel of a fruit than in the center.

5. Plant foods provide _____ concentrated sources of minerals than animal foods.

6. Strict vegetarians may have a _____ mineral-rich diet than people who eat foods from animal sources.

7. Processed foods often have _____ mineral value than whole foods.

8. Fresh fruits and vegetables, whole grains, meat, poultry, and dairy products have _____ mineral value than fats, sugars, and refined flour.

9. Most adults absorb _____ than half of the minerals consumed in their diets.

10. Getting _____ of a mineral than the body requires can interfere with the absorption of other minerals.

11. Problems caused by mineral excesses are _____ often due to the use of supplements than food sources.

12. A diet that is too high in fiber can result in _____ mineral absorption.

13. The use of caffeine and other diuretics results in _____ urine output, thereby increasing the loss of minerals through excretion.

14. The body can absorb _____ calcium and phosphorus in the presence of vitamin D.

15. Eating foods high in vitamin C can result in _____ absorption of iron.

16. The body becomes _____ able to absorb many minerals during times of increased need.

17. Vitamins are _____ stable than minerals.

18. Vegetables that are soaked have _____ mineral content than those that are washed quickly.

19. Cooking methods that require little water promote _____ mineral retention than methods that require a lot of water.

20. Using cooking juices in a dish gives it _____ minerals.

Backtrack
Through Chapter 9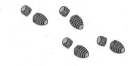

Activity E	**Name** _____
Chapter 9	**Date** _____ **Period**_____

Provide complete answers to the following questions and statements about minerals.

Recall the Facts

- -

1. What is another name for a macromineral and how much of it is needed in the diet? _____
   _____

2. List three functions of calcium other than building strong bones and teeth. _____
   _____
   _____

3. Other than middle-aged women, what group of people is at risk of bone loss due to hormonal changes?
   _____

4. Why is excess phosphorus a problem? _____
   _____

5. A. Name three results of prolonged magnesium deficiency. _____
   _____

   B. Name two results of severe magnesium toxicity. _____
   _____

6. What mineral is found in high concentrations in hair, nails, and skin and produces a distinctive odor when burned? _____
   _____

7. What three minerals help regulate the fluid balance inside and outside the body cells? _____
   _____

8. List three symptoms of potassium deficiency. _____
   _____

9. What are the two forms of iron in food and which one is more easily absorbed? _____
   _____

10. At what times is adequate zinc intake most important? _____
    _____

11. What does an enlarged thyroid gland indicate? _____
    _____

(Continued)

Chapter 9   Minerals: Regulators of Body Functions

12. What can be the result of a selenium deficiency? _____
_____

Interpret Implications

13. What are three problems that are more likely to be experienced by aging people who had inadequate calcium intake during their youth? _____
_____

14. How do sodium and potassium help maintain the proper pH of body fluids? _____
_____

15. Why do females ages 14 through 50 need more iron than males? _____
_____

16. How can excess zinc in the diet affect the body's use of other minerals? _____
_____

17. How can fluoridated drinking water affect the health of a community? _____
_____
_____

Apply & Practice

18. Your father has been diagnosed with hypertension. His doctor has advised him to reduce the sodium in his diet. Your whole family has agreed to modify their sodium intake to help support your father. How would you go about reducing the sodium in your diet? _____
_____
_____

19. You have been experiencing muscle cramps, loss of appetite, and constipation. What do you suspect the problem might be? _____
What would you do about it? _____
_____
_____

20. What are five steps you can take to be sure you are eating a mineral-rich diet? _____
_____
_____
_____
_____

Water: The Forgotten Nutrient 10

Water Crossword

Activity A

Chapter 10

Name _____

Date _____ Period_____

Across

2. A liquid in which substances can be dissolved is a _____.
5. Water outside the cells is _____cellular. (prefix)
8. This contains water to help lubricate food as you swallow it.
10. Water serves as a medium for _____ reactions.
12. A substance that reduces friction between surfaces is a _____.
15. A person who has an abnormal loss of body fluids is said to be _____.
16. A substance that increases urine production is a _____.
19. _____ water has been enhanced with specific nutrients or supplements intended to aid or improve health or energy outcomes.

Down

1. Regularly drinking excessive amounts of water can lead to water _____.
3. Body fluids that contain water are saliva, blood, digestive juices, urine, perspiration, and _____.
4. Water helps remove body wastes through exhaled water vapor, urine, feces, and _____.
6. This body tissue is about 75 percent water.
7. This body tissue is 20 to 35 percent water.
9. This is a lubricant for your eyes.
11. Body fluids that regulate body temperature are perspiration and _____.
13. Water is a _____product of nutrient metabolism. (prefix)
14. Kidneys form this when they draw water and wastes from the blood.
17. Water inside the cells is called _____cellular. (prefix).
18. Water determines the shape, size, and firmness of a(n) _____.

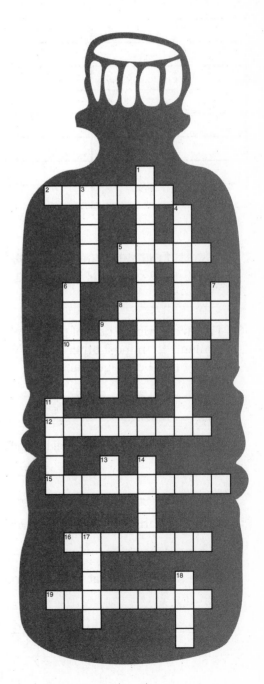

Examining Your Water Needs

Name _____

Date _____ Period _____

Use this beverage diary to record your fluid consumption for 24 hours. (Remember to record your amounts in ounces.) Use Appendix D in the text to find the percentage of each beverage that is water. List this percentage in the third column. Next, for each beverage, find the ounces of water by multiplying the amount consumed by the percentage of water. Record this amount in the fourth column. Then, find the total ounces of water consumed by adding the ounces of water in each beverage. Write this number in the total box. Finally, answer the questions at the bottom of the page.

Beverage	Amount (oz.)	Percent Water	Ounces Water
		Total (oz.)	

1. How did the total ounces of water you consumed compare to the recommended adequate intake for 14- to 18-year-olds of 80 to 112 ounces (2 ½ to 3 ½ quarts) total water? _____
   _____

2. Foods contribute part of the body's needed water. Fruits and vegetables provide higher water contents than most other foods. Name four foods with a high water content that you ate on the day of this beverage diary. _____
   _____
   _____

3. Describe your activity level on the day of this beverage diary. _____
   _____

4. How does an increased activity level affect water needs? _____
   _____

5. Write three goals that will help you improve your water consumption. _____
   _____
   _____

"Water Under the Bridge"

Name _____

Date _____ Period_____

You may have heard people use the expression "water under the bridge" when talking about past experiences. This implies that since the experience is in the past, it is best to forget it. Another way to look at past events is as learning experiences. Read the following mini-cases. In the spaces provided, tell what the teen in each case could learn to avoid similar situations in the future.

Case Situation 1

Sharon had been working in her grandmother's garden for over an hour. She was thirsty, so she quickly drank a quart of ice water from the thermos her grandfather brought. Sharon soon developed a pounding headache. She had to go inside and lie down.

_____

_____

_____

Case Situation 2

When he was sick with the flu, Sean went all day without eating or drinking. He had no appetite and very little thirst. By the end of the day, he was extremely weak and his fever had increased. When his father called the doctor, the first advice he received was to give Sean plenty of fluids.

_____

_____

_____

Case Situation 3

Harold was a member of the school wrestling team. During the summer he gained five pounds. He had just one week to lose the added weight before the new season began. He decided to fast, exercise, and take diuretics in order to reduce his water weight as quickly as possible.

_____

_____

_____

Case Situation 4

When she first started her running routine, Helen noticed she was always thirsty. She did not like the taste of her tap water. Instead, she drank one soft drink after another to try to quench her thirst. No matter how many soft drinks she drank, she was still thirsty. Finally, she decided to buy gallon jugs of bottled water, which seemed to work better.

_____

_____

_____

Drinking Water—The Undiluted Truth

Name _____

Date _____ Period _____

For each statement, write *T* in the blank if the statement is true or *F* in the blank if the statement is false. Then answer the questions at the bottom of the page.

_____ 1. The more expensive bottled waters are better for you than tap water.

_____ 2. Tap water often contains minerals that affect its taste.

_____ 3. Water from private wells may contain microorganisms.

_____ 4. Bottled water contains minerals that enhance your health.

_____ 5. Public water sources are tested and required to meet federal health standards.

_____ 6. Bottled water must meet higher standards for purity than public drinking water.

_____ 7. Private well water can be tested for contaminants.

_____ 8. Bottled water is always safer than tap water.

_____ 9. The presence of iron and sulfur deposits in water causes it to be hazardous.

_____ 10. Fortified water comes from special wells located in specific geographic locations.

Think It Over...

11. Do you prefer bottled water, filtered water, or tap water? Explain. _____

_____

_____

12. Why do you think bottled water is so popular? _____

_____

_____

13. Why do you think many people use filtration pitchers or systems? _____

_____

_____

14. Is bottled water worth the cost? Why? _____

_____

_____

15. Are water filtration pitchers and systems worth the cost? Why? _____

_____

_____

Backtrack
Through Chapter 10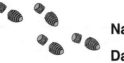

Provide complete answers to the following questions and statements about water.

Recall the Facts

1. The body contains approximately how many gallons of water? _____

2. For most adults, what percentage of body weight is water? _____

3. What are the vital functions of water? _____

    _____

    _____

4. What is an electrolyte and what does it do? _____

    _____

5. Give an example to illustrate that some foods are higher in water content than some beverages.

    _____

6. What is the average amount of water loss per person each day? _____

7. What are the four paths by which water leaves the body? _____

    _____

8. What does a diuretic do? Give two examples of diuretics. _____

    _____

9. Why is it dangerous to lose 10 percent or more of your body weight through water losses? _____

    _____

10. What is considered to be a healthy urine output? _____

11. State three reasons some people buy bottled water instead of drinking tap water. _____

    _____

    _____

12. Give examples of nutrients or supplements commonly used in fortified waters. _____

    _____

(Continued)

Interpret Implications

13. Explain why water is sometimes considered the most essential nutrient. _____
_____
_____

14. What does water do in its important role as a solvent? _____
_____
_____

15. Explain how water helps regulate body temperature in both cold and warm weather conditions.
_____
_____

16. Explain how the water balance inside and outside the cells remains fairly constant. _____
_____
_____

17. Why do pregnant and lactating women have increased water needs? _____
_____
_____

Apply & Practice

18. Your doctor has advised you to increase your water intake. Which beverages would you choose
to help you meet this goal and which would you avoid? Explain. _____
_____
_____
_____

19. You have become ill with a stomach virus, which has left you unable to eat. Your doctor tells you
it is okay to wait until you feel hungry before you eat again. The doctor says you should continue
to drink plenty of fluids even if you are not thirsty. Is this good advice? Why or why not? _____
_____
_____
_____

20. Name four specific ways you can include more water in your diet. _____
_____
_____
_____

The Life Cycle

Activity A

Chapter 11

Name _____

Date _____ Period_____

1. Write the names of the life-cycle stages discussed in this chapter.

   Stage: _____

   Stage: _____

   Stage: _____

   Stage: _____

   Stage: _____

   Stage: _____

2. Explain why nutrition experts subdivide some stages of the life cycle into more specific life-stage groups. _____

   _____

3. What are two lifestyle choices that can impact nutritional needs during the life cycle? _____

   _____

   _____

4. Explain why individuals in the same life-cycle stage may have different nutritional needs.

   _____

   _____

   _____

5. Why is it important to understand the relationship between life cycle and nutritional needs?

   _____

   _____

Nutrition During Pregnancy and Lactation

Name _____

Date _____ Period_____

Complete the following statements about changing nutritional needs during pregnancy and lactation.

_____ 1. A name for producing breast milk is _____.

_____ 2. Care that is given during a woman's pregnancy to reduce the risk of complications to both mother and fetus is called _____.

_____ 3. Women who become pregnant when they are 10 percent or more below healthy weight have a greater risk of having a _____ baby, or a baby that is too small.

_____ 4. A _____ baby is one that is born before the 37th week of pregnancy.

_____ 5. Each one-third of pregnancy (about 13 to 14 weeks) is called a _____.

_____ 6. Pregnant women need to consume extra _____ to build fetal tissue and support changes in their own bodies. Many already get more than enough of this nutrient.

_____ 7. An increased amount of the vitamin _____ is needed to aid in the development of the baby's brain and spinal cord.

_____ 8. Pregnant women who are vegetarians need to eat fortified foods or take supplements containing vitamin _____. This vitamin occurs naturally only in animal foods.

_____ 9. Pregnant women must consume enough _____ to prevent losses from their bones.

_____
_____
_____
_____ 10. Four minerals besides calcium for which a woman's needs increase during pregnancy are _____, _____, _____, _____.

_____ 11. Along with extra nutrients, pregnant women need additional _____ from the food they eat to supply energy to support fetal development.

_____ 12. Average weight gain during pregnancy for a woman of normal weight is between _____ and _____ pounds.

_____ 13. In addition to vitamin and mineral supplements, lactating women need increased amounts of protein, calories, and _____.

_____ 14. The craving for and ingestion of nonfood materials such as clay, soil, or chalk is called _____.

_____ 15. In pregnant women, _____ has been linked to having low-birthweight babies. It causes babies to be deprived of oxygen, which endangers their health.

_____ 16. Any substances in the mother's blood pass into the bloodstream of the fetus through the blood vessels in the _____.

_____ 17. When a lactating woman uses a drug, it can be secreted in her _____ and affect her baby as well.

_____ 18. _____ is a set of disorders that includes brain damage, retarded growth, and irregular facial features. It is often present in infants whose mothers drank alcohol during pregnancy.

Feeding an Infant

Name _____

Date _____ Period_____

Complete the following activities related to infant feeding.

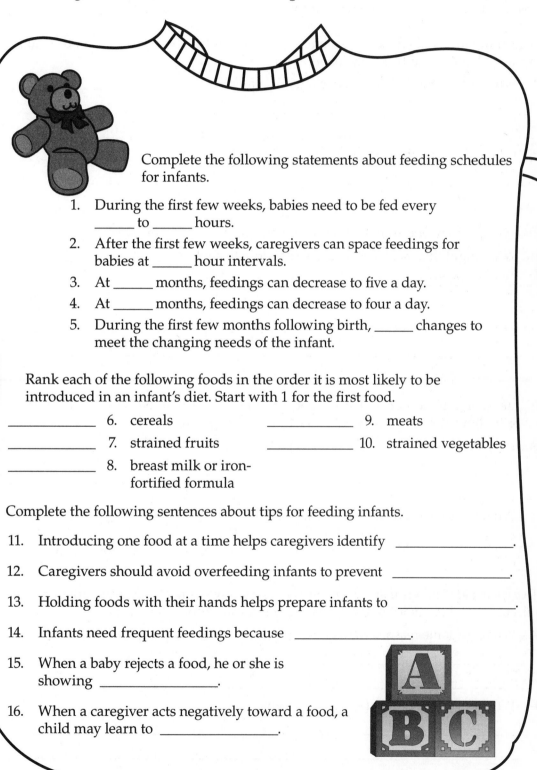

Complete the following statements about feeding schedules for infants.

1. During the first few weeks, babies need to be fed every _____ to _____ hours.

2. After the first few weeks, caregivers can space feedings for babies at _____ hour intervals.

3. At _____ months, feedings can decrease to five a day.

4. At _____ months, feedings can decrease to four a day.

5. During the first few months following birth, _____ changes to meet the changing needs of the infant.

Rank each of the following foods in the order it is most likely to be introduced in an infant's diet. Start with 1 for the first food.

_____ 6. cereals   _____ 9. meats

_____ 7. strained fruits   _____ 10. strained vegetables

_____ 8. breast milk or iron-
              fortified formula

Complete the following sentences about tips for feeding infants.

11. Introducing one food at a time helps caregivers identify _____.

12. Caregivers should avoid overfeeding infants to prevent _____.

13. Holding foods with their hands helps prepare infants to _____.

14. Infants need frequent feedings because _____.

15. When a baby rejects a food, he or she is showing _____.

16. When a caregiver acts negatively toward a food, a child may learn to _____.

Sticky Situations

A number of eating problems can arise when children reach the toddler stage. Read these "sticky situations" and answer the questions that follow.

1. Fifteen-month-old Sarah ate a few bites of her spaghetti. Then she smeared the sauce on the tray of the high chair and threw the noodles on the floor.

   A. Why do you think Sarah is such a messy eater? _____

   _____

   _____

   B. What advice would you give her caregiver? _____

   _____

   _____

2. One-year-old Theodore choked twice during his lunch of beanie weanies and a sliced banana.

   A. Why might this meal have caused Theodore to choke? _____

   _____

   _____

   B. What advice would you give his caregiver? _____

   _____

   _____

3. Eighteen-month-old Ronald usually eats his lunch in front of the TV while his mom watches her favorite show. Ronald usually eats very little before getting down to play.

   A. Why do you think Ronald eats so little? _____

   _____

   _____

   B. What advice would you give his mother? _____

   _____

   _____

4. Two-year-old Cathy is usually a good eater. Recently she has not wanted to eat her food. She has rejected even her favorites. Cathy's caregiver doesn't know what to do.

   A. What are some reasons why Cathy may have become a picky eater? _____

   _____

   _____

   B. What advice would you give her caregiver? _____

   _____

   _____

Serving Up Teen Nutrition

Activity E

Chapter 11

Name _____

Date _____ Period_____

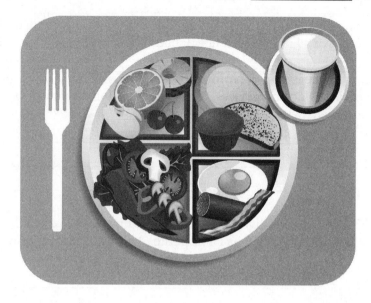

Fill in the blanks to complete these statements about teen nutrition.

1. _____ is the period of life between childhood and adulthood.
2. _____ is the time during which a person reaches sexual maturity.
3. Most adolescents experience a period of rapid physical growth that is known as a _____.
4. Body _____ changes during adolescence as females develop a layer of fatty tissue and males develop more lean body mass.
5. A teen's daily calorie needs are _____ than they were in late childhood.
6. The average teen female needs _____ calories per day.
7. Teen males need more calories than teen females because they have more _____.
8. An 18-year-old male needs _____ more calories per day than a female of the same age.
9. Teens need to replenish supplies of energy and nutrients at _____ intervals throughout the day.
10. _____ eating patterns can cause teens to be tired, irritable, drowsy, and distracted.
11. Breakfast should provide _____ of a teen's daily nutrient needs.
12. Teens should choose fast foods in _____ because they are high in sugar, fat, and sodium.
13. Some teens who do not consume enough iron may develop _____.
14. Females need more iron than males due to _____.
15. Weight problems of teens include overweight, underweight, and eating _____.
16. Inadequate calcium intake during the teen years can affect bone _____.
17. Too much sugar during the teen years can cause dental _____.
18. A high-fat diet during the teen years can increase the risk of _____ disease in later life.

Chapter 11   Nutrition Across the Life Span

Advice for Adults

Name _____

Date _____ Period_____

Read the case situations involving adult nutrition advice. In the space provided, describe the advice as good or bad and explain why. For any instance of bad or incomplete advice, offer a suggestion.

1. Mary tells her doctor she does not like milk and has always avoided dairy products to help keep her weight down. The doctor advises her to begin taking a calcium supplement before she approaches the age of menopause.

   _____

   _____

   _____

2. Jenny's mother is 75 years old and lives alone in the country. Lately, she has been eating very little and losing weight. She says she has no appetite. A friend advised Jenny to bring her mother home for the weekend and try to make her eat before things get worse.

   _____

   _____

   _____

3. Pat notices her husband has been gaining weight in the past few weeks. His pants are too tight in the waist, and he is using new holes in his belts. She advises him to pay more attention to what he is eating. She reminds her husband it's better to keep weight off than to try to lose it later.

   _____

   _____

   _____

4. George has been having problems with constipation. He mentioned this to his brother, who advised him to eat a high-fiber diet and drink lots of fluids.

   _____

   _____

   _____

5. Since his wife died, Bob has had to cook his own meals. He has found cooking for one to be challenging. His daughter asked him to try lunches offered at the Sunny Senior Center.

   _____

   _____

   _____

Backtrack
Through Chapter 11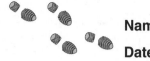

Activity G

Chapter 11

Name _____

Date _____ Period_____

Provide complete answers to the following questions and statements about nutrition throughout the life cycle.

Recall the Facts

1. Which stages of the life cycle have you already completed? _____
   _____

2. How does gender determine the amounts of nutrients a person needs? _____
   _____

3. Why do a woman's nutritional needs change during pregnancy? _____
   _____
   _____

4. When a mother chooses to breast-feed, what nutrients does she need in even greater amounts than when she was pregnant? _____
   _____

5. What harmful effects can FAS have on a baby? _____
   _____

6. During what stage is growth more rapid than at any other stage? _____

7. What is generally considered to be the ideal food for infants and why? _____
   _____
   _____

8. What amount of food from the grains group is suitable for a two-year-old toddler? _____
   _____

9. The childhood stage of the life cycle includes which ages? _____

10. List four healthful snacks parents can provide for children. _____

11. What are two major causes of childhood weight problems? _____
    _____

12. How does a growth spurt affect nutritional needs? _____
    _____

13. List the names and age ranges of the four stages into which nutrition experts divide adulthood.
    _____

(Continued)

Interpret Implications

14. How can drugs used by a mother harm her baby during pregnancy and lactation? _____

    _____

15. Describe how teen pregnancy causes special problems not seen in the pregnancies of adult
    women. _____

    _____

    _____

16. How can healthful eating increase a person's ability to perform well in school or on the job?

    _____

17. Briefly describe three ways nutritional needs change after age 50. _____

    _____

    _____

Apply & Practice

18. Plan a day's menus for a teen using the nutritional information from the chapter.

Breakfast	Lunch	Snack	Dinner

19. List two tips to consider when planning meals for someone in each of the following stages of the
    life cycle.

    A. pregnancy and lactation _____

    _____

    B. infancy _____

    _____

    C. toddlerhood _____

    _____

    D. childhood _____

    _____

    E. adolescence _____

    _____

    F. adulthood _____

    _____

The Energy Balancing Act

12

Calorie Calculations

Activity A

Chapter 12

Name _____

Date _____ Period _____

Show the calculations you use to solve each of the following problems involving energy input and output.

1. The Nutrition Facts panel on a box of macaroni and cheese tells you a serving provides 230 calories. The panel shows a serving provides 90 calories from fat. A serving provides 9 grams of protein and 26 grams of carbohydrate. How many calories come from protein and carbohydrate?

2. Your physician advises you to limit your fat intake to no more than 30 percent of your daily calories. Suppose your daily diet included 260 grams of carbohydrates, 75 grams of fat, and 60 grams of protein. Are you following your doctor's advice? Explain.

3. A broiled chicken sandwich weighs 248 grams and provides 540 calories. A double bacon cheeseburger weighs 159 grams and provides 460 calories. Which of the two fast foods is more calorie dense?

4. What would be the basal energy needs per day of a man who weighs 175 pounds?

5. Refer to Figure 12-7 in the text. Use the average in each range of calories. Estimate the number of calories Carlos burned through physical activity from 7:00 AM to 12:00 noon on Saturday morning. Carlos rose at 7:00 for an early morning run. He returned at 8:00, had breakfast, and read the paper until 9:00. Then he showered, dressed, washed dishes, and cleaned the kitchen until 10:00. From 10:00 to noon, he raked leaves.

6. Stephanie burns about 2,400 calories per day. Approximately how many of these calories are for each of the following needs: basal metabolism, physical activity, and thermic effect of food?

Health Hangs in the Balance

Name _____

Date _____ Period_____

Read the following statements about energy imbalance. Circle *T* if the statement is true. Circle *F* if the statement is false.

T   F   1. Going on a weight-loss diet is an example of creating an intentional energy deficiency.

T   F   2. Energy deficiency occurs when energy output is less than energy intake.

T   F   3. Energy deficiencies may be caused by poverty, famine, illness, or dieting.

T   F   4. When there is an energy deficiency, the body draws first on fatty tissue to meet its needs.

T   F   5. The stored form of glucose from carbohydrates for use by nonmuscle tissue is liver glycogen.

T   F   6. Glycogen stores will be depleted within two to three hours after the body begins to draw on them for energy.

T   F   7. Weight loss occurs as the body draws on fatty tissue for energy.

T   F   8. The nervous system uses only fat as a fuel source.

T   F   9. The body can convert fat into glucose for use as a fuel source.

T   F   10. The body can easily make glucose from amino acids to feed the nervous system without any health consequences.

T   F   11. Breaking down muscle proteins causes a rapid weight loss due to loss of body fluids.

T   F   12. Changing fatty acids into ketone bodies is the body's way of limiting muscle deterioration when carbohydrates are not available.

T   F   13. A buildup of ketone bodies in the bloodstream is a sign of good health.

T   F   14. Ketosis changes the acid-base balance of the blood.

T   F   15. Low-carbohydrate diets are recommended by most nutritionists.

T   F   16. A weight-loss diet needs to include adequate amounts of carbohydrates to prevent damage to body protein tissues.

T   F   17. Energy excess occurs when energy output is less than energy intake.

T   F   18. Excess calories are stored as adipose tissue.

T   F   19. An excess of 2,400 calories in the diet leads to one pound of stored body fat.

T   F   20. The amount of weight a person gains within a given time depends on the degree of energy excess.

T   F   21. Just a small daily energy excess can result in a number of added pounds of body fat over a period of years.

T   F   22. The more excess fat a body has, the greater the risks for health problems.

Evaluate Your Weight

Activity C

Chapter 12

Name _____

Date _____ Period_____

Complete the following exercises to help you evaluate your weight and compare various weight evaluation tools.

Body Mass Index

1. What is your height in inches? _____

2. What is your weight in pounds? _____

3. Calculate your body mass index by completing the following equations.

   A. $\underset{\text{height}}{\underline{}} \times \underset{\text{height}}{\underline{}} = \underset{\text{height}^2}{\underline{}}$

   B. $\underset{\text{weight}}{\underline{}} \div \underset{\text{height}^2}{\underline{}} = \underset{\text{X}}{\underline{}}$.

   C. $\underset{\text{X}}{\underline{}} \quad \underset{\text{constant}}{\underline{703}} = \underset{\text{BMI}}{\underline{}}$

4. What does your BMI indicate about the status of your weight? _____

   _____

5. Do you think body mass index is an appropriate weight evaluation tool for you? _____
   Explain why. _____

   _____

Body Composition Measurement

6. Do a pinch test by grasping the skin on the back of your upper arm halfway between your shoulder and elbow. Pinch this fold of skin between your thumb and forefinger. Be sure to grasp only the fat, not the muscle. What is the distance between your thumb and forefinger? _____

   _____

7. What does this indicate about your body composition? _____

   _____

8. Is the pinch test an appropriate body composition evaluation tool for you? _____
   Explain why. _____

Location of Body Fat

9. Locate your natural waist by tying a length of string around your body about 3 inches above your navel. Bend over as though to touch your toes to cause the string to settle at the smallest place, which is your natural waist. Use a tape measure to measure the circumference of your waist. _____

10. What is the goal for waist circumference for men? _____ for women? _____ Does your waist circumference meet the goal for your gender? _____

11. Use a tape measure to measure your maximum hip circumference. _____ Divide your waist circumference by your hip circumference to determine your waist-to-hip ratio. _____

12. What is the goal for waist-to-hip ratio for men? _____ for women? _____ Does your waist-to-hip ratio meet the goal for your gender? _____

13. Are you a fully grown adult? _____ Keep in mind that these methods for evaluating location of body fat are applicable only for fully grown adults.

In Balance

Name _____

Date _____ Period_____

Use the clues provided to identify terms related to energy balance. Write one letter in each space. Use the circled letters to name the two sides of the energy balance equation at the bottom of the page.

1. The concentration of energy in a food is referred to as __ __ __ __ __ __ __ __Ⓞ__ __ __ __ __.

2. An adult with a body mass index below 18.5 is defined as __Ⓞ__ __ __ __ __ __ __ __ __ __.

3. The energy required to complete the processes of digestion, absorption, and metabolism is called the __ __ __ __ __ __ __ __Ⓞ__ __ __ __ __ __ __ __ __ __ __.

4. A measure of the body's resting energy expenditure based on data that is collected four hours after eating or physical activity is called the __ __ __ __ __ __ __ __ __ __ __ __ __ __ __ __ Ⓞ__ __ __.

5. __ __ __ __ Ⓞ__ __ is the ability to do work.

6. A __ __ __ __ __ __ __ __ __Ⓞ __ __ __ __ __ __ __ __ is an activity that requires a lot of sitting.

7. The amount of energy required to support the operation of all internal body systems except digestion is known as __ __ __ __ __ __ __ __ __ __ __ __ __Ⓞ__ __.

8. A process that measures body fat by measuring the body's resistance to a low-energy electrical current is __ __ __ __ __ __ __ __ __ __ __ __ __ __ __ __ __ __ __Ⓞ__ __.

9. Compounds formed from fatty acids the nervous system can use for energy when carbohydrates are not available are called __ __ __ __ __Ⓞ __ __ __ __ __ __ __ __.

10. A test in which the thickness of a fold of skin is measured to estimate the amount of subcutaneous fat is called a __ __ __Ⓞ__ __ __ __ __ __ __ __ __.

11. An adult with a body mass index of 30 or more is defined as __ __Ⓞ__ __.

12. An adult with a body mass index of 25 to 29.9 is defined as __ __ __Ⓞ__ __ __ __ __ __ __.

13. Body weight that is specific to gender, height, and body frame size and associated with health and longevity is called __ __ __ __ __ __ __ __ __ __ __ __ __ __ __ __Ⓞ__ __.

14. A calculation of body weight and height used in federal guidelines to define underweight, healthy weight, overweight, and obesity is __ __ __Ⓞ__ __ __ __ __ __ __ __ __ __ __ __ __ __.

15. The percentage of different types of tissues in the body, such as fat, muscle, and bone, refers to __ __ __ __ __ __ __ __ __ __Ⓞ__ __ __ __ __ __ __.

16. Fat that lies underneath the skin is called __ __ __ __ __Ⓞ__ __ __ __ __ __ __ __ __ __ __ __.

17. The average calories needed to maintain energy balance in a healthy person of a certain age, gender, weight, height, and level of physical activity is called __ __ __ __ __ __ __ __ __ __ __ __ __ __ __ __ __ __ __ __ __ __ __ __ __ __Ⓞ.

The Energy Balance Equation

__ __ __ __ __ __ __ __ __ __ __ = __ __ __ __ __ __ __ __ __ __

Backtrack
Through Chapter 12

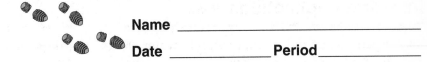

Activity E

Chapter 12

Name _____

Date _____ Period_____

Provide complete answers to the following questions and statements about energy balance.

Recall the Facts

- -

1. What type of energy is stored in food? _____

2. From what three nutrient groups does the body obtain food energy? _____
   _____

3. What three factors account for the calories you expend each day? _____
   _____

4. Which internal body system is not included in the amount of energy designated for basal metabolism? _____
   _____

5. What hormone regulates basal metabolism? _____

6. What three aspects of physical activity cause an increase in energy needs? _____
   _____

7. Name five activities that would be described as sedentary. _____
   _____

8. What term refers to the energy required to get the energy from food? _____

9. What is the first step the body takes to meet its energy needs when there is not enough food energy available? _____
   _____

10. Without stating a BMI range, describe what it means to have a healthy body weight. _____
    _____

11. Why are younger women sometimes described as "pear-shaped" while older people are often described as "apple-shaped"? _____
    _____

12. What percentage of fat in the body is subcutaneous fat? _____
    _____

(Continued)

Interpret Implications

13. Explain why foods that are high in water are low in calorie density and foods that are high in fats are high in calorie density. _____

_____

_____

14. Why would a 150-pound member of the women's swim team burn more calories than her 110-pound teammate swimming at the same pace? _____

_____

15. Why might someone intentionally create an energy imbalance in his or her body? _____

_____

16. How can a small daily energy excess affect health? _____

_____

17. Explain why the location of body fat appears to affect health. _____

_____

_____

Apply & Practice

18. Use the Estimated Energy Requirements chart in Appendix C to find your recommended energy intake. How does that amount compare with your recommended intake ten years ago, five years ago, five years from now, and ten years from now? Why do you think the amounts change?

_____

_____

_____

19. Explain factors that might cause your BMR and RMR to differ from that of an inactive, five-foot two-inch, 50-year-old woman. _____

_____

_____

_____

20. The 14-year-old Swanson twins, Jake and Janet, are each five feet three inches tall and weigh 130 pounds. What is the twins' body mass index? _____

_____

Use the body mass index-for-age percentile graphs in Appendix F to determine the weight status of each twin. How do they compare? Explain your answer.

_____

_____

Weigh the Risks

Activity A

Chapter 13

Name _____

Date _____ Period_____

The list below contains health risks of being overweight and risks of being underweight. Each risk is identified by a letter. If a risk is associated with being underweight, write the letter in the pan of the scale labeled "underweight." If the risk is associated with being overweight, write the letter in the "overweight" pan. Note that some risks belong in both pans. Be prepared to support your answers. In the space provided, write a paragraph about the risk of most interest to you. Summarize ways to "tip the scales in your favor."

A. cancer

B. discrimination

C. fatigue

D. heart disease

E. hypertension

F. inability to stay warm

G. inadequate nutrient stores

H. irregular menstruation

I. low self-esteem

J. osteoarthritis

K. pregnancy complications

L. respiratory problems

M. surgical complications

N. type 2 diabetes

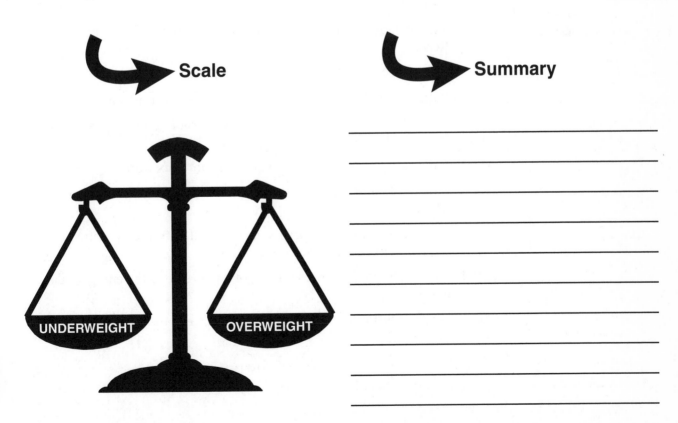

Scale

Summary

UNDERWEIGHT   OVERWEIGHT

Facts and Factors

Name _____

Date _____ Period_____

Examine the following statements about factors affecting weight status. If the statement is true, write *true* in the blank. If the statement is false, change the underlined word or phrase to make the statement true. Write the correct word or phrase in the blank.

_____ 1. <u>Weight</u> management means attaining healthy weight and keeping it throughout your life.

_____ 2. <u>Heredity</u> affects the shape of your body.

_____ 3. The size of your bones and the location of fat stores on the body are <u>inherited</u> traits.

_____ 4. Your <u>heredity</u> affects your basal metabolic rate.

_____ 5. A family history of obesity <u>does</u> necessarily mean you will be obese.

_____ 6. Weight management may be <u>easier</u> for a person who inherited genes that lean toward obesity.

_____ 7. Parents <u>can</u> greatly influence a child's eating habits.

_____ 8. Parents can plan their children's meals and snacks around appropriate portions of <u>nutritious</u> foods.

_____ 9. Teens have <u>more</u> control over what they eat than children do.

_____ 10. Many teens form habits of eating foods that are <u>low</u> in fat and calories.

_____ 11. Eating habits <u>may</u> be influenced by schedules, peers, and weight concerns.

_____ 12. <u>Work and family</u> obligations sometimes negatively affect eating patterns.

_____ 13. Adults who commute to work often eat <u>at home</u>.

_____ 14. Situations that trigger you to eat are called environmental <u>cues</u>.

_____ 15. Social settings and time of day are examples of <u>hereditary</u> factors that influence weight status.

_____ 16. Being aware of when and why you eat <u>is not</u> important.

_____ 17. Examples of <u>environmental</u> factors include depression, boredom, fear, tension, and loneliness.

_____ 18. People <u>can</u> look for appropriate ways to deal with their emotions while following a nutritious diet.

_____ 19. Physical activity influences the "calories <u>in</u>" side of the energy balance equation.

_____ 20. An <u>active</u> lifestyle can lead to an energy excess and unwanted weight gain.

The Math of Weight Loss

Nate is a moderately active 16-year-old. He typically has 30 to 60 minutes of daily activity. He knows he has developed a pattern of unhealthy eating habits in the past year and as a result has gained weight. Answer the following questions to help Nate achieve a healthy weight. Show your work.

1. What are Nate's approximate daily energy needs in calories? (Use the "Daily Food Plan" on ChooseMyPlate.gov or the Estimated Energy Requirements in Appendix C.)

2. Nate kept a food diary for one week and estimates his daily calorie intake is 3,200 calories. How many surplus calories does this intake represent?

3. If Nate's eating habits and physical activity remain the same, what is the possible weight gain over one year? (Round to nearest whole number.)

4. Nate sets a goal to lose 12 pounds in 10 weeks. How many pounds per week weight loss does this represent? Is this a safe goal?

5. By how many calories per day must Nate reduce his intake to achieve his goal?

6. Since Nate is still growing, what are other ways he could lose weight without reducing his intake of nutritious foods?

Believe It or Not?

A new weight loss center has just opened in town. Operators of the center claim to have the best and latest methods for weight loss. Evaluate each claim posted on the storefront below. In the space provided at the bottom of the page, write *Believe it* next to the claims you believe and *Not* next to the claims you do not believe. Write a brief statement to support each response.

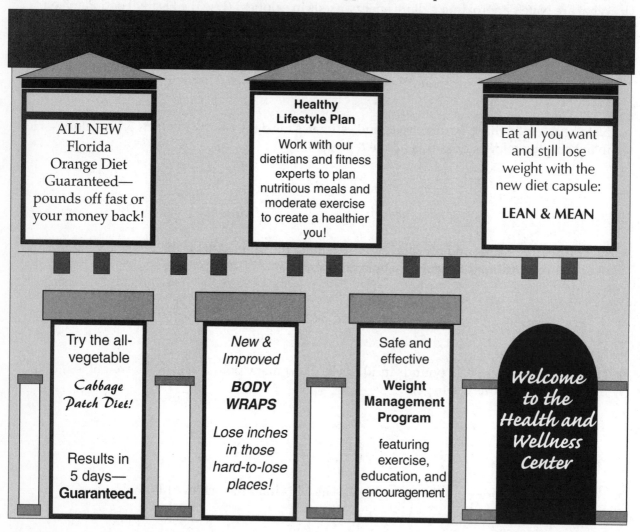

1. Florida Orange Diet

2. Healthy Lifestyle Plan

3. Lean & Mean

4. Cabbage Patch Diet

5. Body Wraps

6. Weight Management Program

In the Driver's Seat

When it comes to weight management, it seems everyone has advice to give. Read each piece of advice below. In the blanks, write *GA* for each piece of good advice and *BA* for each piece of bad advice. Then in the space provided, explain why the advice is good or bad. When it comes to weight management, you are in the driver's seat—you are in control of your own food intake and energy balance.

_____ 1. Think of food as the enemy and self-denial as the goal.

_____

_____ 2. See a doctor before you begin a weight loss program.

_____

_____ 3. Think of losing weight as managing intake, not as dieting.

_____

_____ 4. Read any weight loss plan you are considering carefully and thoroughly.

_____

_____ 5. The best diets are those that allow you to take off pounds quickly.

_____

_____ 6. Choose a diet that is as close to your food preferences as possible.

_____

_____ 7. The all-carrot diet is a good choice because carrots have a lot of vitamins.

_____

_____ 8. A good diet should allow you to eat out without social discomfort or embarrassment.

_____

_____ 9. Avoid diets that are based on the use of pills.

_____

_____ 10. Fasting is well-named because it is the fastest and best way to lose weight.

_____

_____ 11. To lose weight, cut down on vegetables and whole-grain foods.

_____

_____ 12. Lose weight slowly to avoid health risks.

_____

_____ 13. Replace high-fat snacks with fresh fruits.

_____

_____ 14. Keep a food diary to help identify problem eating behaviors.

_____

_____ 15. Two or three square meals a day are better than five or six smaller meals.

_____

(Continued)

_____ 16. A good way to cut calories is to skip breakfast.

_____

_____ 17. Choose steamed or broiled, not fried, foods when you eat out.

_____

_____ 18. Drink a glass of water before a meal so you will not feel so hungry.

_____

_____ 19. Weigh yourself only once or twice a week.

_____

_____ 20. Always clean your plate.

_____

_____ 21. Consider going to see a registered dietitian to get counseling about weight loss.

_____

_____ 22. Diet pills are not addictive as long as you follow the recommended dosage.

_____

_____ 23. Substitute low-calorie ingredients in the recipes you prepare at home.

_____

_____ 24. Increase your physical activity to help curb short-term hunger.

_____

_____ 25. Use a smaller plate so your portions of food do not look so small.

_____

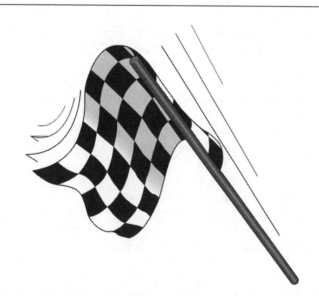

Backtrack
Through Chapter 13

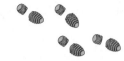

Activity F

Chapter 13

Name _____

Date _____ Period _____

Provide complete answers to the following questions and statements about healthy weight management.

Recall the Facts

1. What does weight management mean? _____
   _____

2. What percentage of people in the United States are overweight or obese? _____

3. Why is reducing obesity a national health goal in the United States? _____

4. List three reasons being underweight can be a problem. _____
   _____

5. List three types of factors that influence weight status. _____

6. Name three environmental cues that affect eating habits. _____
   _____

7. What energy deficit in calories is needed to lose one pound of body fat? _____

8. Does a higher level of activity increase or decrease a person's daily calorie needs? _____

9. What is the difference between a fad diet and a crash diet? _____
   _____

10. What is weight cycling? _____
    _____

11. In general, how much weight can a person safely lose in one week? _____

12. If a person is trying to gain weight, why should he or she avoid drinking extra fluids just before mealtime?
    _____

Interpret Implications

13. List two disadvantages of liquid diet programs. _____
    _____

14. What causes a person to gain weight? _____
    _____
    _____

(Continued)

15. To what extent does the FDA protect consumers from false weight-loss claims? _____

_____

_____

16. What are the dangers of fasting? _____

_____

_____

17. Suggest five ways an underweight person might work toward safe weight gain. _____

_____

_____

_____

Apply & Practice

- -

18. While being overweight is almost always seen as a health concern, being underweight is commonly overlooked as a health concern. Why do you think this is? What, if anything, can be done to change this? _____

_____

_____

_____

19. This chapter describes several ways to change eating habits—keeping a food diary, using activities to manage emotions, finding new responses to cues, writing a habit change contract, and setting up a points system. If your doctor advised you to lose or gain weight, which approach would work best for you and why?

_____

_____

_____

_____

20. After reading about recent discoveries about the role of leptin and ghrelin in appetite regulation and energy expenditure, one parent reacted by saying, "Perhaps this explains the current increase in childhood obesity." What would be your response to this parent?

_____

_____

_____

_____

_____

Eating Disorders 14

Read the Warning Signs

Name _____

Date _____ Period_____

Read the following list of characteristics and health risks associated with various eating disorders. If an item describes anorexia nervosa, write *AN* in the blank. If an item describes bulimia nervosa, write *BN* in the blank. If an item describes binge-eating disorder, write *BED* in the blank. Some items may describe more than one eating disorder.

_____ 1. A cycle of bingeing and purging is repeated at least twice a week.

_____ 2. A sense of power is derived from controlling weight.

_____ 3. Amenorrhea develops among females.

_____ 4. Baggy clothes may be used to help hide an overly thin body.

_____ 5. Behavior is hidden from others.

_____ 6. Denial becomes an obstacle to treatment.

_____ 7. Dieting becomes a life-threatening obsession.

_____ 8. Eating patterns are recognized as abnormal.

_____ 9. Excessive exercise may be used to prevent weight gain.

_____ 10. Fear of weight gain is intense.

_____ 11. Feeling cold is a common complaint.

_____ 12. Feelings of guilt about overeating are common.

_____ 13. Forced vomiting may be used to prevent weight gain.

_____ 14. Health problems may result from excess weight.

_____ 15. Huge amounts of food are eaten uncontrollably.

_____ 16. No steps are taken to prevent weight gain.

_____ 17. Personality is highly achievement oriented.

_____ 18. Throat glands may become swollen.

_____ 19. Tooth enamel may be destroyed by stomach acids.

_____ 20. Weight-loss programs are often not completed.

Help for Eating Disorders

Name _____

Date _____ Period _____

In the space provided, briefly describe the role each of the following people may play in the treatment of eating disorders.

1. medical doctor _____

   _____

   _____

2. psychologist _____

   _____

   _____

3. registered dietitian _____

   _____

   _____

4. exercise specialist _____

   _____

   _____

5. family members _____

   _____

   _____

6. friends _____

   _____

   _____

7. support group members _____

   _____

   _____

8. family therapists _____

   _____

   _____

What role must a person with an eating disorder play in his or her treatment?

_____

_____

_____

Media Pressure to Be Thin

Activity C

Chapter 14

Name _____

Date _____ Period_____

Some of the theories about the causes of eating disorders are briefly described in the text. According to one theory, the social pressure to be thin can cause people to form unhealthful eating habits. The media—advertisements, television programs, magazines, the Internet, and other media—are powerful sources of social pressure. For this activity, you will find and analyze messages from various media sources about thinness and body image.

Advertisement

Find an advertisement that portrays thinness as desirable. Staple the ad to this page. Then answer the following questions about the ad.

1. Where did the advertisement come from? _____

2. What product or service is being sold by the ad?

   _____

3. What type of person is the ad trying to influence. How do you know this?

   _____

   _____

   _____

4. Describe how the ad portrays thinness as desirable or exerts pressure to be thin.

   _____

   _____

   _____

Television

Find a television show that portrays thinness as desirable. Answer the following questions about the program.

1. Name of television show: _____

   _____

2. Describe who you think is the intended audience for this program and why.

   _____

   _____

   _____

3. Describe how the show portrays thinness as desirable or exerts pressure to be thin.

   _____

   _____

   _____

(Continued)

Magazine

Find a magazine that portrays thinness as desirable. Then answer the following questions about the magazine.

1. Name of magazine: _____

2. Summarize content of the magazine. _____

    _____

    _____

3. Describe who you think is the intended audience (readers) of this publication and why. _____

    _____

    _____

    _____

4. Describe how the magazine portrays thinness as desirable or exerts pressure to be thin.

    _____

    _____

    _____

Website

Find a website that portrays thinness as desirable. Then answer the following questions about the website.

1. Name of the website: _____

2. Describe the content of the website.

    _____

    _____

    _____

3. Describe who you think is the intended audience of the website and why.

    _____

    _____

    _____

4. Describe how the website portrays thinness as desirable or exerts pressure to be thin.

    _____

    _____

    _____

Backtrack
Through Chapter 14

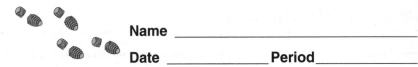

Activity D

Chapter 14

Name _____

Date _____ Period_____

Provide complete answers to the following questions and statements about eating disorders.

Recall the Facts

- -

1. What are the three most common eating disorders? _____

   _____

2. To what two groups of people are eating disorders most common? _____

3. List five traits that people who develop eating disorders often share. _____

   _____

   _____

4. Name four methods used by people with bulimia to purge. _____

   _____

5. What are three emotions that often accompany binge-eating disorder? _____

   _____

6. Name one major source of social pressure to be thin. _____

7. What three types of family patterns have been associated with the development of eating
   disorders? _____

   _____

   _____

8. What three medical problems comprise the female athlete triad? _____

   _____

9. What are the chances that a person with anorexia nervosa will recover completely if given proper
   treatment? _____

   _____

10. What is outpatient treatment? _____

11. What is the goal of counseling in treating binge-eating disorder? _____

    _____

12. What role would a registered dietitian play in treating someone with an eating disorder? _____

    _____

(Continued)

Interpret Implications

13. What motivates people with anorexia nervosa to keep dieting? _____

_____

_____

14. Why are people with bulimia sometimes harder to identify than people who have anorexia nervosa? _____

_____

15. Why is the risk of developing an eating disorder higher during the teen years? _____

_____

16. How can verbal skills and stress management techniques help someone who has anorexia nervosa? _____

_____

17. How can people recovering from bulimia avoid having relapses? _____

_____

Apply & Practice

18. Suppose you are a member of a sports team at school. The coach repeatedly tells team members they must watch their weight if they want to compete. What could you privately say to the coach about his or her influence on the development of eating disorders among team members? _____

_____

_____

19. How could you help a family member with an eating disorder feel comfortable with members of a health care team? _____

_____

_____

20. What would you do if you believed your friend had bulimia nervosa? _____

_____

_____

Assessing Activity Goals

Activity A

Chapter 15

Name _____

Date _____ Period _____

Provide honest answers to the following questions about your physical activity habits. Based on your answers, determine which of the three main goals for physical activity you are closest to meeting—good health, total fitness, or peak athletic performance.

1. What physical activities are part of your daily routine? _____

   _____

   _____

2. What household tasks do you do regularly? _____

   _____

   _____

3. Do you participate in any regular exercise programs? If so, describe.

   _____

   _____

4. Are you involved in any training programs to develop specific sports skills? Describe the programs and what skills you are developing.

   _____

   _____

5. How much time do you spend each day engaged in moderate-intensity aerobic activities (such as brisk walking, bike riding, or raking leaves)? _____

6. How many days a week do you engage in vigorous-intensity aerobic activities (such as basketball, swimming, or running)? _____

7. How many days a week do you engage in muscle-strengthening activities? _____

8. How many days a week do you engage in bone-strengthening activities? _____

9. Which physical activity goal—good health, total fitness, or peak athletic performance—are you closest to meeting? _____

   _____

10. Suggest ways you can meet each of the other two physical activity goals.

    _____

    _____

Physical Activity Crossword

Activity B

Chapter 15

Name _____

Date _____ Period_____

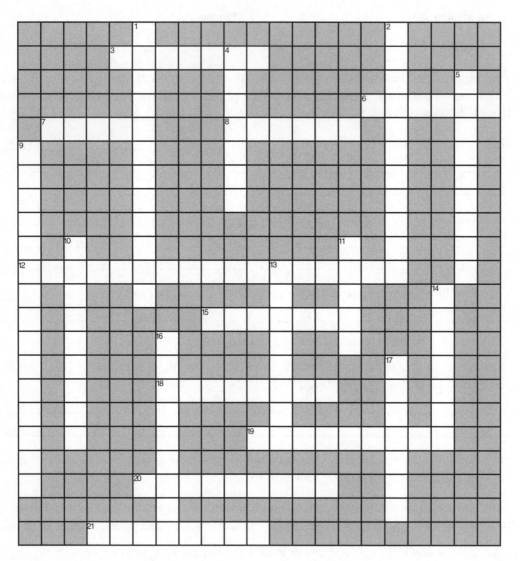

(Continued)

Nutrition & Wellness for Life Student Workbook   Copyright by Goodheart-Willcox Co., Inc.

Across

3. The position of your body when standing or sitting.
6. *Aerobic* means with _____.
7. The quickness with which you are able to complete a motion.
8. This heart rate zone is the range of heartbeats at which the heart muscle receives its best workout.
12. The body's _____ fitness describes its ability to take in oxygen and carry it through the blood to body cells.
15. Your ability to keep your body in an upright position while standing or moving.
18. How long an exercise session lasts.
19. How hard you exercise.
20. Activities in which your muscles use oxygen faster than your heart and lungs can deliver it.
21. The ability of the muscles to move objects.

Down

1. The ability to integrate the use of two or more parts of the body.
2. The ability to move your joints through a full range of motion.
4. Your _____ heart rate is the speed at which your heart muscle contracts when you are sitting quietly.
5. Another name for pulse rate.
9. A level of physical condition in which all body systems function together efficiently.
10. How often you exercise.
11. The ability to do maximum work in a short time; requires strength and speed.
13. Your _____ time is the amount of time it takes you to respond to a signal.
14. The ability to change body position with speed and control.
16. The ability to use a muscle group over and over without becoming tired.
17. Your _____ heart rate is the highest speed at which the heart muscle is able to contract.

Physical Activity for Life—Easy as 1-2-3

Activity C

Chapter 15

Name _____

Date _____ Period_____

Figuring out physical activity levels for children, teens, and adults is as easy as remembering 1-2-3. Complete the spaces in these *Physical Activity Guidelines for Americans* using a "1," "2," or "3" in each space. Then check your answers against the *Guidelines* found in Chapter 15 of your textbook. Finally, for #8, highlight and list any guidelines you are currently not following and need to add to your daily routine.

Adults (18 to 64 years old)

1. Should do _____ hours and _____0 *minutes a week* of moderate-intensity, or _____ hour and _____5 *minutes a week* of vigorous-intensity aerobic physical activity, or an equivalent combination of moderate- and vigorous-intensity aerobic physical activity. Aerobic activity should be performed in episodes of at least _____0 minutes, preferably spread throughout the week.

2. Additional health benefits are provided by increasing to 5 the number of *hours a week* of moderate intensity aerobic physical activity, or _____ hours and _____0 *minutes a week* of vigorous intensity physical activity, or an equivalent combination of both.

3. Should also do muscle-strengthening activities that involve all major muscle groups performed on _____ or more *days per week*.

Children and Adolescents (6 to 17 years old)

4. Should do _____ hour or more of physical activity *every day*.

5. Most of the _____ hour or more of physical activity each day should be either moderate- or vigorous-intensity aerobic activity, and should include vigorous-intensity physical activity at least _____ *days per week*.

6. Part of the daily physical activity should include muscle-strengthening activity on at least _____ *days per week*.

7. Part of the daily physical activity should include bone-strengthening activity on at least _____ *days per week*.

8. Are there guidelines that you are currently not following? If so, write those guideline(s) below and list ways you can incorporate each into your daily routine. _____

_____

_____

_____

_____

_____

_____

_____

Backtrack
Through Chapter 15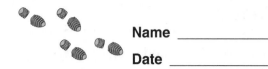

Activity D

Chapter 15

Name _____

Date _____ Period_____

Provide complete answers to the following questions and statements about physical activity.

Recall the Facts

- -

1. List the three main goals for physical activity. _____
   _____

2. How much moderate activity is required per day for a person between the ages of 6 and 17 to achieve good health? _____

3. How can exercise improve posture? _____
   _____

4. Exercise can lower the risk of developing some diseases. Name four. _____
   _____

5. List the five components of physical fitness. _____
   _____

6. Give three examples of aerobic activity. _____

7. Give three examples of anaerobic activity. _____

8. List three activities that can build muscle endurance. _____
   _____

9. What is body composition? _____
   _____

10. Give an example to demonstrate how speed can help in daily living. _____
    _____
    _____

11. Name four keys to a successful exercise program. _____
    _____

12. Name two signs you are working out too hard. _____

13. What are the three phases of a workout session? _____
    _____

(Continued)

Interpret Implications

14. Why should people of all body types and sizes consider the benefits of physical activity for weight management?

_____

15. Explain why anaerobic activities do not increase cardiorespiratory fitness. _____

_____

_____

16. Why does a slower heartbeat indicate increased fitness? _____

_____

_____

17. How does exercise affect cholesterol levels? _____

_____

Apply & Practice

18. Write one fitness goal for yourself. Then list the steps you could take to achieve this goal.

_____

_____

_____

_____

_____

_____

19. Make a list of physical activities you enjoy. Then make a second list of physical activities you have never tried. Place a check by those you *think* you might enjoy. _____

_____

_____

_____

_____

_____

20. Calculate your maximum heart rate and your target heart rate zone. Show your work. _____

_____

_____

_____

_____

_____

Eating for Sports Performance 16

Ask an Athlete

Activity A　　　　　　　　　　　**Name** _____

Chapter 16　　　　　　　　　　　**Date** _____ **Period** _____

Use the questions below as a guide for interviewing an athlete of your choice. Record the athlete's responses, but not his or her name. Be prepared to discuss the benefits and/or dangers of the performance practices you find.

1. What type of sports do you perform? _____

2. What foods do you eat or avoid just before an event? Why? _____

   _____

3. What steps do you take to increase your endurance? _____

   _____

4. What foods do you eat for energy? _____

   _____

5. What do you prefer to drink before, during, and after a sporting event? _____

   _____

6. Have you ever tried to gain or lose weight to improve your athletic performance? If so, what
   changes did you make? _____

   _____

   _____

7. Have you ever taken any type of pill or drink to try to enhance athletic performance? If so, what
   were the results? _____

   _____

   _____

   Based on your interview, would you classify this athlete as "very conscious," "somewhat
   conscious," or "not very conscious" of eating for sports performance? Explain. _____

   _____

   _____

   Based on what you have learned, suggest two ways the athlete you interviewed could improve
   his or her habits regarding eating for sports performance. _____

   _____

   _____

Analyze This

Activity B

Chapter 16

Name _____

Date _____ **Period**_____

Read a news or feature article about eating for sports performance. The article can come from a current general or fitness-related publication or website. Then complete the following analysis of the article based on what you have learned from this chapter.

1. Title of the article: _____

2. Author(s) of the article: _____

3. If the article appears online, give the website name and the name of the group that created it. Otherwise, give the publication's name, date, and page number(s) of the article. _____

   _____

   _____

4. What is the focus of the article? _____

   _____

   _____

   _____

5. Is the article well written? Why or why not? _____

   _____

   _____

   _____

6. Give an example of how studying the chapter helped you understand the subject presented in the article.

   _____

   _____

   _____

7. Give two examples of new information or ideas you gathered from the article. _____

   _____

   _____

   _____

8. Based on your study of the chapter, did the article seem to be misleading or inaccurate? Explain.

   _____

   _____

   _____

9. Would you recommend this article to a friend? Why or why not? _____

   _____

Forty-Fact Relay

See if you can distinguish facts from falsehoods in this challenging "Forty-Fact Relay." If the statement is true, write the word "True" in the blank. If the statement is false, change the underlined word(s) to make the statement true. Write the corrected word(s) in the blank.

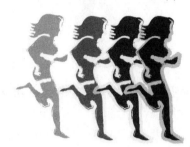

_____ 1. People who weigh more, burn <u>fewer</u> calories during a given activity.

_____ 2. More vigorous activities require <u>more</u> energy than less active sports.

_____ 3. Weight is lost whenever an athlete consumes <u>more</u> calories than he or she burns through exercise.

_____ 4. Athletes need to take in <u>more</u> calories than nonathletes to maintain a healthy body weight.

_____ 5. Fat <u>is not</u> burned for energy during aerobic activity.

_____ 6. <u>Glucose</u> is the body's chief source of energy.

_____ 7. Lactic acid builds up in the muscles from lack of <u>oxygen</u> to break down glucose.

_____ 8. Athletes <u>can</u> train their muscles to improve the use of glucose.

_____ 9. Athletes <u>need</u> vitamin and mineral supplements.

_____ 10. Dried fruits and yogurt shakes <u>are</u> good concentrated sources of energy for athletes.

_____ 11. Carbohydrate loading involves eating a <u>high-protein</u> diet for several days followed by several days of eating a high-carbohydrate diet.

_____ 12. Taking rest days <u>can</u> help athletes build up glycogen stores.

_____ 13. Eating within 30 <u>hours</u> after an activity ends helps the body replenish muscle glycogen.

_____ 14. In recovery, the most important nutrient is a <u>protein</u> with a high glycemic index that enters the bloodstream quickly.

_____ 15. Read <u>ingredient</u> lists if you choose to use recovery drinks.

_____ 16. You need to get adequate <u>sleep</u> to help your body fully recover.

_____ 17. The most critical nutritional need of athletes is <u>fluid</u> intake.

_____ 18. Athletes can see how much water they lose by weighing themselves <u>after</u> events.

_____ 19. Athletes can lose <u>four to six pounds</u> of water weight during an event.

(Continued)

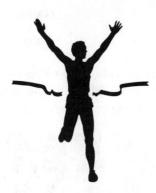

_____ 20. Exercising in humid weather tends to <u>decrease</u> the amount of water lost during exercise.

_____ 21. <u>Fruit juice</u> is the preferred liquid for fluid replacement during athletic events.

_____ 22. Caffeine and alcohol tend to <u>decrease</u> body water loss.

_____ 23. Using salt tablets is a <u>good</u> way to replenish sodium lost by sweating.

_____ 24. Frequent <u>smaller</u> meals are better before performance events.

_____ 25. A good pregame meal should be high in <u>protein</u> and low in fat.

_____ 26. The acceptable level of body fat for female athletes is <u>greater</u> than for male athletes.

_____ 27. Weight lifters <u>strengthen</u> their endurance by avoiding fluids one or two days before an event.

_____ 28. Standard practice for training wrestlers <u>does</u> involve the use of laxatives and emetics to reduce body weight prior to competition.

_____ 29. The best time for athletes to diet is just before <u>competition</u> begins.

_____ 30. <u>Rapid</u> weight loss is the best way to lose unwanted pounds.

_____ 31. Consuming 3,500 fewer calories than are expended results in the loss of <u>one pound of body fat</u>.

_____ 32. Athletes who need to gain weight should increase their intake by 2,500 calories per <u>day</u>.

_____ 33. Athletes who need to gain or lose weight should work with a registered <u>dietitian</u>.

_____ 34. Athletes <u>can</u> trust the claims of many sports performance enhancers.

_____ 35. A planned program of supervised training and nutritious eating is the <u>safest, most effective</u> key to peak athletic performance.

_____ 36. Marathon bicyclists and distance swimmers are examples of <u>endurance</u> athletes.

_____ 37. Athletes <u>cannot</u> usually meet their protein needs without making major diet modifications.

_____ 38. Symptoms of iron <u>overload</u> for athletes include fatigue and breathlessness.

_____ 39. Snacking on foods before you exercise can help to <u>lower</u> your energy levels.

_____ 40. Muscle size <u>can</u> be increased by consuming more calories.

Backtrack
Through Chapter 16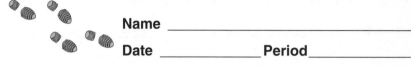

Activity D

Chapter 16

Name _____

Date _____ Period_____

Provide complete answers to the following questions and statements about eating for sports performance.

Recall the Facts

1. List five benefits of sports participation. _____

   _____

2. What has increased the spread of nutrition myths and misinformation among athletes? _____

   _____

3. Where do muscles get the energy needed to fuel activity? _____

   _____

   _____

4. How are the aerobic and anaerobic energy production systems used by the body? _____

   _____

   _____

5. What is lactic acid and how does it affect the body? _____

   _____

6. Why do athletes need to eat a variety of foods that are rich in vitamins and minerals? _____

   _____

7. What problems can occur when athletes practice carbohydrate loading? _____

   _____

8. What are the symptoms of dehydration? _____

   _____

9. How much water is generally lost per hour by sweating during a vigorous workout? _____

10. What fluid intake is recommended by the National Athletic Trainers' Association before, during, and after an athletic event? _____

    _____

    _____

    _____

11. What are some reasons why salt tablets are not recommended to replace sodium lost during physical activity? _____

    _____

(Continued)

12. For most sports events, when should a pregame meal be eaten? _____

13. What can you conclude about claims of performance enhancers that sound too good to be true?

_____

Interpret Implications

14. Explain why the calorie needs of athletes are greater than those of nonathletes. _____

_____

_____

15. Explain what it means when an athlete "hits the wall." _____

_____

_____

16. Explain how percentage of body fat affects athletic performance. _____

_____

_____

17. List one type of performance aid sometimes used by athletes. Explain why this performance aid can have harmful effects and suggest a healthful alternative. _____

_____

_____

_____

18. Explain why an athlete might be concerned with gaining or losing weight. What additional considerations do athletes have when trying to lose, gain, or maintain body weight? _____

_____

_____

Apply & Practice

19. Plan a menu for a pre-event lunch for a weight lifter. _____

_____

_____

_____

_____

20. Plan a menu for a pregame breakfast for a hockey player. _____

_____

_____

_____

Maintaining Positive Social and Mental Health

17

Applying Maslow's Hierarchy

Activity A

Chapter 17

Name _____

Date _____ Period_____

On the pyramid diagram, write the name for each level of Maslow's hierarchy of human needs. Then on the two lines provided to the right of each level, write two examples for each type of need. Finally, answer the questions on the next page.

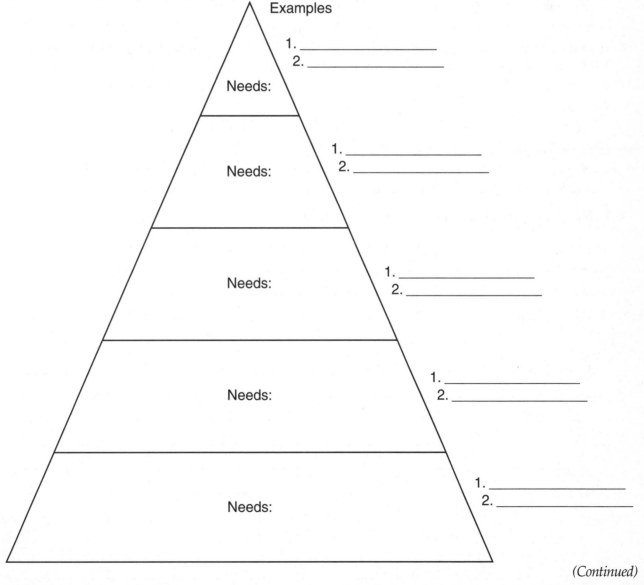

Examples

Needs: 1._____ 2._____

Needs: 1._____ 2._____

Needs: 1._____ 2._____

Needs: 1._____ 2._____

Needs: 1._____ 2._____

(Continued)

1. If a person cannot address physical needs, how does this affect the person's ability to meet self-actualization needs? _____

_____

_____

_____

_____

_____

2. Explain how safety and security needs can be threatened by living in a dangerous neighborhood. How can a person feel more safe in this type of environment? _____

_____

_____

_____

_____

_____

3. If a person's love and acceptance needs are unmet in childhood, how can this affect the person? What can he or she do to fill these unmet needs? _____

_____

_____

_____

_____

_____

4. Explain how people can satisfy their esteem needs. _____

_____

_____

_____

_____

5. Why is addressing a self-actualization need important? _____

_____

_____

_____

_____

_____

Communication Snapshot

Activity B

Chapter 17

Name _____

Date _____ **Period** _____

You will be given parts of conversations between students. For each person's communication, circle whether it was ineffective or effective. Use the "Rationale" section to explain why. Then, where needed, suggest what the person could have done differently to improve communication.

1. Brian knew his debate teammates wouldn't like what he had to say. He'd thought about what to say and said it just like he planned. "I know our competition is next week, and you have all been counting on me to be there. We've had two resignations at Dad's store, so now I have to work that day. I'm really sorry."

   Ineffective   Effective

   Rationale: _____

   _____

   Suggestion: _____

   _____

2. Without pausing to think, Gerald blurted out, "Deserter!" After that, he refused to speak to Brian any more that day.

   Ineffective   Effective

   Rationale: _____

   _____

   Suggestion: _____

   _____

3. Looking down at her notebook, Susan moaned, "What a mess!"

   Ineffective   Effective

   Rationale: _____

   _____

   Suggestion: _____

   _____

4. Samantha asked, "Are you saying you've made every effort possible to find someone to work in your place?"

   Ineffective   Effective

   Rationale: _____

   _____

   Suggestion: _____

   _____

(Continued)

5. Rolling his eyes toward the ceiling, Josh said, "It must have been a tough choice for you."

   Ineffective   Effective

   Rationale: _____

   _____

   Suggestion: _____

   _____

6. Tamika mumbled, "Whatever…"

   Ineffective   Effective

   Rationale: _____

   _____

   Suggestion: _____

   _____

7. Jeremy said, "I've listened to what you said. I'm disappointed, but I understand your dilemma. You must be feeling really bad."

   Ineffective   Effective

   Rationale: _____

   _____

   Suggestion: _____

   _____

8. With a sad look on her face, Patricia said, "Do you think we care if you mess this up for us? We didn't want you to go anyway."

   Ineffective   Effective

   Rationale: _____

   _____

   Suggestion: _____

   _____

Dear Peacemaker

Name _____

Date _____ Period_____

Pretend you write a column called "Dear Peacemaker" for a local newspaper. The column gives readers advice about positive conflict resolution. Use the space provided to answer the following letters from your readers about their conflict concerns.

Dear Peacemaker,

I am disgusted with my friend for being so selfish. Whenever we hang out together, we always have to do what he wants and go where he wants—you get the picture. For once, I wish we could do something I like! But I'm afraid to say anything. I don't want to make him mad or hurt his feelings.

"Doormat in Decatur"

Dear Doormat,

_____

_____

_____

_____

_____

_____

Peacemaker

Dear Peacemaker,

I have a big problem with my mom. She always treats me like I am still a three-year-old. When I try to tell her about it, she gets very upset and gives me all kinds of grief. She brings up all the times I was late coming in, got a ticket for speeding, didn't clean my room—you name it! All I want is to be treated like the young adult I am!

"Feeling Grown in Grovetown"

Dear Grown,

_____

_____

_____

_____

_____

_____

Peacemaker

Dear Peacemaker,

I thought brothers were supposed to be close. I can't wait until my brother leaves home for college. He stays on my case about everything—like borrowing his new cap without asking and playing my music too loud when he's studying! He is so unreasonable. No one could please a brother who is that picky! Why do I even bother? I have my own life to live.

"No Bother Brother"

Dear Brother,

_____

_____

_____

_____

_____

_____

Peacemaker

Dear Peacemaker,

My friend and I are not getting along very well lately. She made me really mad, but I didn't tell her. I just got madder and madder on the inside. Then, one day, I blew up at her and said lots of things I really didn't mean. Now she doesn't want to be my friend anymore. Is there anything I can do to make this situation better?

Snapdragon

Dear Snapdragon,

_____

_____

_____

_____

_____

_____

Peacemaker

Teams Work

Name _____

Date _____ Period_____

Take a closer look at the advantages of teamwork by examining the TEAM acronym- "Together Everyone Accomplishes More!" Answer the questions related to each word in the acronym in the spaces provided.

Together

1. What does it mean to cooperate? _____

_____

2. What does it mean to compromise? _____

_____

3. Specifically, how can members of a team encourage one another? _____

_____

Everyone

4. Why is each person's job important to the success of the team? _____

_____

5. How can members respond if one team member is not doing his or her share? _____

_____

6. How can members treat others as valued members of the team? _____

_____

Accomplishes

7. How should groups establish common goals? _____

_____

8. How can groups be assured team goals will be reached? _____

_____

More!

9. Why are teams often more effective than individuals? _____

_____

10. Why are complex problems best addressed by groups? _____

_____

Countdown to Mental Health

Activity E

Chapter 17

Name _____

Date _____ Period_____

Read each question below and check the appropriate column. Then answer the questions at the bottom of the page.

	Usually	Sometimes	Never
Do you...			
1. surround yourself with people who are supportive?			
2. find role models to serve as good examples?			
3. connect with encouraging friends?			
4. avoid negative thoughts about yourself?			
5. protect your physical health?			
6. eat nutritious foods?			
7. get plenty of rest?			
8. get regular physical activity?			
9. avoid harmful substances?			
10. devote enough time and energy to each of your roles?			
11. actively work on your listening, as well as speaking, skills?			
12. become proactive when choosing your circle of friends?			

13. For how many responses did you check the "Usually" column? _____

14. For how many responses did you check the "Never" column? _____

15. What do you think this indicates about your mental health? _____

_____

16. Select one item you think you could improve. Write the number here. _____

17. List three goals you could set to address this area. _____

_____

_____

_____

Managing Myself

Name _____

Date _____ Period_____

Prepare a self-management plan for making a positive behavioral change in your life. Follow the steps outlined below and fill in the chart.

List your strengths   _____ _____   _____ _____
List your improvements needed in order of importance   ( )_____ ( )_____   ( )_____ ( )_____
Clarify your goal   Express your most-needed improvement as a specific goal.   _____   _____
List the alternatives for achieving your goal   Indicate advantages and disadvantages of each option.   _____   _____   _____   _____   _____
Make a choice and act on it   Choose the alternative that seems best. Write it below. Act on it.   _____   _____
Evaluate outcomes   Analyze the results of your actions.   _____   _____   _____

Backtrack
Through Chapter 17

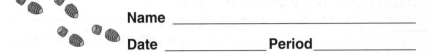

Activity G

Chapter 17

Name _____

Date _____ Period_____

Provide complete answers to the following questions and statements about social and mental health.

Recall the Facts

- -

1. What is a hierarchy? _____

2. Where do the closest and most lasting social relationships occur for most people? _____

3. What other group of people in your social circle serves as a valuable source of self-discovery?
   _____

4. What type of communication involves the use of spoken or written words? _____

5. What type of communication sends messages without using words? _____

6. For the following "you" message, give a corresponding "I" message: "You make me so mad when you say you will call but don't." _____
   _____

7. What is assertiveness? _____
   _____

8. Name five characteristics of effective teams. _____
   _____
   _____

9. What are characteristics of good friends? _____
   _____
   _____

10. What five main types of roles do most people have? _____
    _____

11. List three questions that can help you evaluate the outcomes of a self-management plan. _____
    _____
    _____
    _____

12. What does burnout mean? _____
    _____

13. When social and mental health problems are too great to be solved with self-help techniques, what should a person do? _____

(Continued)

　　Chapter 17　Maintaining Positive Social and Mental Health　　125

Interpret Implications

14. Explain Maslow's rationale for the theory that lower-level needs must be met before a person can address higher-level needs. Give an example to support your explanation. _____

_____

_____

_____

15. Explain the link between self-awareness and social health. _____

_____

16. Explain the influential role a caregiver can have in a child's social development. What implications does this have for parents who are selecting a child care arrangement for their children? _____

_____

_____

17. Explain the difference between assertive and aggressive. _____

_____

_____

18. Explain the difference between self-concept and self-esteem. _____

_____

_____

Apply & Practice

19. Describe in detail someone you know who has positive social and mental health. _____

_____

_____

_____

20. Recall interactions you have observed between people today. List two actions you saw that built self-esteem and two actions you saw that diminished it. _____

_____

_____

_____

_____

_____

Stress and Wellness

18

Do Not Stress Out!

Activity A

Chapter 18

Name _____

Date _____ **Period** _____

Complete the puzzle by filling in the appropriate terms in the statements below.

1. Minor daily stresses that produce tension are called _____ _____.
2. Someone with a type A _____ tends to be driven to achieve goals.
3. Divorce is an example of a _____-_____ _____, or a major stressor that can greatly alter a person's lifestyle.
4. A technique of focusing on involuntary bodily processes in order to control them is called _____.
5. A reaction in which your body is gathering its resources to conquer danger is a _____ response.
6. The inner agitation you feel when you are exposed to change is _____.
7. A reaction in which your body is gathering its resources to escape to safety is a _____ response.
8. _____ muscle relaxation is a relaxation technique that involves slowly tensing and then relaxing different groups of muscles.
9. Harmful stress is called _____ _____.
10. Your internal conversations about yourself and the situations you face are called _____-_____.
11. A source of stress is a _____.
12. Stress that motivates you to accomplish challenging goals is _____ _____.
13. A person or group of people who can provide you with help and emotional comfort is your _____ _____.
14. Another name for negative stress is _____.

Stress Metaphors

Activity B

Chapter 18

Name _____

Date _____ Period_____

Consider the following metaphor about stress:

Stress is like a rubber band...when life pulls at you, you stretch and give, and stretch and give, and hope that you don't POP!

Use the space below to write your own original metaphor for stress.

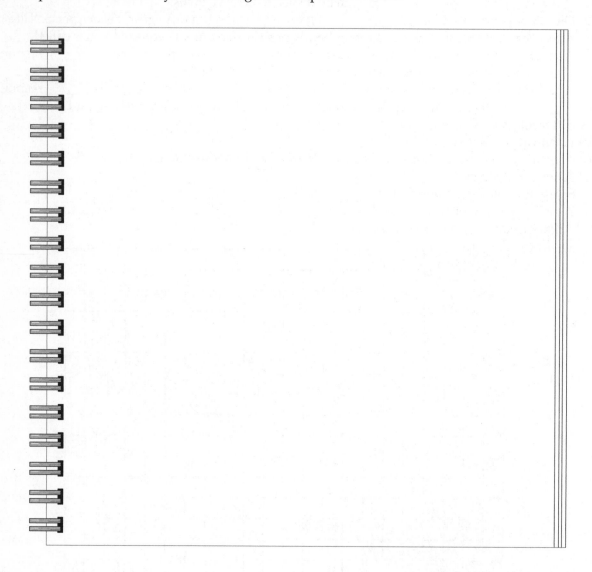

Good Stress/Bad Stress

Name _____

Date _____ Period _____

Read the situations below and identify each type of stress as either *positive* or *negative*. For each situation of positive stress, identify one good result that could occur. For each situation of negative stress, identify one bad result that could occur.

1. The air was charged with the excitement and anticipation of the crowd. The team ran onto the field for the big game. The crowd cheered, and Jeff, the quarterback, felt a quiver of nervousness race up his spine.

   Type of Stress: _____

   Result: _____

   _____

2. Kara had studied thoroughly for the midterm. As the teacher began to hand out the tests, Kara felt a momentary sense of uncertainty. She took a deep breath and told herself, "Relax, you know this. Just be cool."

   Type of Stress: _____

   Result: _____

   _____

3. Andrew's father is an alcoholic. Andrew never knows when his dad will lose his temper. His dad is angrier these days, and his drinking causes him to miss work. Andrew dreads going home, not knowing what he will find.

   Type of Stress: _____

   Result: _____

   _____

4. Rebecca keeps hearing rumors of impending layoffs at work. Not knowing whether or not she will lose her job is beginning to wear on her nerves. Rebecca feels anxious and edgy.

   Type of Stress: _____

   Result: _____

   _____

5. Justice is worried. Lately he has noticed physical symptoms that may indicate a serious health problem. The problem runs in his family. He's afraid to go to the doctor, wondering if his worst fears will be realized.

   Type of Stress: _____

   Result: _____

   _____

6. Kendra tutors a friend several days a week after school. After several weeks, Kendra misses having the time to do her own homework, participate in after-school activities, and hang out with other friends. Her friend has grown to rely on Kendra and does not want the tutoring to end.

   Type of Stress: _____

   Result: _____

   _____

The Pileup Effect

Name _____

Date _____ Period_____

The diagram below illustrates how one stressor leads to a series of other stressors, creating a pileup effect. Once the stress builds so high, it becomes overwhelming. Look at the completed diagram and answer the questions.

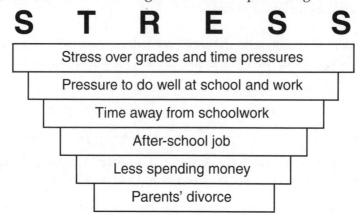

S T R E S S

Stress over grades and time pressures

Pressure to do well at school and work

Time away from schoolwork

After-school job

Less spending money

Parents' divorce

1. What was the core cause of the stress pileup? _____

2. Explain in your own words how the core cause might have caused poor grades as a result of the pileup effect.

   _____

   _____

Now create your own diagram of the pileup effect. At the base of the pyramid, write an example of a core stressor. You may use either a real or imaginary example. At each level, write an example that illustrates how stressors can pile up on one another.

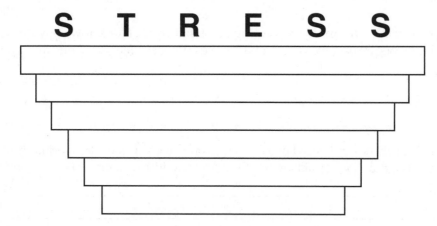

S T R E S S

3. List three examples of what a person at the bottom level of the pyramid could have done to alleviate stress.

   _____

   _____

4. How can a person's support system help in alleviating the pileup effect?

   _____

5. Why is it important to deal with smaller stressors before stress has a chance to pile up?

   _____

Straight Talk on Stress

Activity E

Chapter 18

Name _____

Date _____ Period_____

If the statement is true, write the word *true* in the blank. If the statement is false, change the underlined word(s) to make the statement true. Write the correct word(s) in the blank.

_____ 1. The body goes through three stages when it responds to stress—alarm, <u>fight</u>, and exhaustion.

_____ 2. The alarm stage contains both emotional and <u>mental</u> responses.

_____ 3. During the alarm stage, a person's heart rate and blood pressure are likely to <u>increase</u>.

_____ 4. <u>Narrowing</u> of eyes and tensing of muscles are signs the body is preparing to conquer danger or escape.

_____ 5. During the <u>alarm</u> stage, a person's stress level may start to subside and the muscles begin to relax.

_____ 6. During the <u>exhaustion</u> stage, you may feel tired and unable to concentrate.

_____ 7. Prolonged tension in one area of your life <u>can</u> spill over into other areas.

_____ 8. Chronic stress <u>can</u> lead to physical illness.

_____ 9. Stress can cause physical reactions as stress hormones are released into your <u>brain</u>.

_____ 10. Physical reactions to stress include rapid heartbeat, <u>retention</u> of glucose by the liver, and release of fat cells into the bloodstream.

_____ 11. Increases in heart rate and blood pressure <u>can</u> strain your heart.

_____ 12. Extra fat released into the bloodstream during periods of stress <u>can</u> build up in your arteries.

_____ 13. The immune system's defenses can be <u>heightened</u> during periods of stress.

_____ 14. During times of stress, your increased level of mental activity can keep you from <u>falling asleep</u>.

_____ 15. When stress hormones are active, your body treats food digestion as a <u>high</u> priority.

_____ 16. Stress <u>can</u> be a factor in the development of weight problems and eating disorders.

_____ 17. Your reactions to stress <u>can</u> compromise your nutritional status, and in turn, produce outcomes that compound your stress.

_____ 18. <u>Physical</u> effects of stress include irritability and worry.

_____ 19. Factors that determine how you respond to stressors include <u>heredity</u>, experience, and outlook.

_____ 20. Someone with a type A personality is often more <u>relaxed about</u> stressful events than someone with a type B personality.

Friends in Need

Name _____

Date _____ Period_____

For each scenario below, provide advice to the person under stress. Suggest one positive way the person can manage the stress he or she feels.

1. Shannon is usually a very cheerful person. Lately she has been moody. She has been complaining about headaches and lack of energy. For the past few days, Shannon has not wanted to be around her friends.

   _____

   _____

   _____

2. Theo has been under a lot of stress. He found out his mother has cancer. He has not shared his feelings and fears with his friends. He doesn't want to "bring them down." The school counselor asked to meet with Theo, but Theo managed to find a schedule conflict to avoid the meeting. He just doesn't want to talk about the situation.

   _____

   _____

   _____

3. Holden had waited in a long line of cars to enter the parking lot. Just as it was his turn, another driver cut in front of him and entered the lot first. As Holden inched forward toward the entrance to the parking lot, the "Lot Full" sign appeared.

   _____

   _____

   _____

4. Stacey had always had a hard time with math problems. As she sat down to do her homework, she told herself, "I'm no good at this. I always get more problems wrong than right. I don't know why I even try."

   _____

   _____

   _____

5. Jonathan starts working on assignments early. He loses interest, though, and never seems to finish them until the night before they are due. Sometimes he has to stay up all night, but he always gets them done. Jonathan concludes he works better under pressure.

   _____

   _____

   _____

6. Since she heard about her parents' upcoming divorce, Marita has been depressed. She has stopped taking her daily jog and her appetite has suffered. From the circles under her eyes, it appears she hasn't been sleeping either.

   _____

   _____

   _____

Backtrack
Through Chapter 18

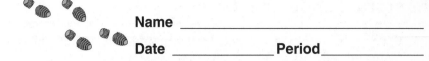

Activity G

Chapter 18

Name _____

Date _____ Period _____

Provide complete answers to the following questions and statements about stress and wellness.

Recall the Facts

1. What feeling usually accompanies stress? _____

2. What are the two types of stress? _____

3. How can negative stress reduce your effectiveness? _____
_____

4. How can positive stress produce good results? _____
_____

5. Is feeling lonely a life-change event or a daily hassle? Why? _____
_____

6. Is moving to a new city a life-change event or a daily hassle? Why? _____
_____

7. What is the flight or fight response? _____
_____

8. Give an example to illustrate each stage of the body's response to stress. _____
_____
_____

9. List three serious physical health problems that may result from the effects of stress. _____
_____

10. Name three types of effects stress can have on your physical health. _____
_____

11. List five techniques that can help you manage stress. _____
_____
_____

12. List five suggestions for preventing stress by addressing its root causes. _____
_____
_____
_____

13. What is biofeedback? _____
_____

(Continued)

Interpret Implications

14. Give one example of a physical stressor and one example of an emotional stressor. Offer a suggestion for alleviating each of these stressors. _____

_____

_____

_____

15. Give an example that illustrates how families in crisis may experience large amounts of stress.

_____

_____

16. Explain how a person can use biofeedback to manage stress. _____

_____

_____

17. Explain how a person's support system (or lack of support) can affect his or her ability to handle stress effectively.

_____

_____

18. If a person feels stress due to lack of time, would cutting out leisure activities be a good way to manage this stress? Explain. _____

_____

_____

Apply & Practice

19. Select a common stressor in the lives of teens. Write a paragraph describing the stressor, its causes, and ways teens can prevent or cope with the stress it creates. _____

_____

_____

_____

_____

20. Write a brief paragraph describing the connection between a person's attitude and his or her experience of stress. Give examples you have observed in real-life situations._____

_____

_____

_____

_____

_____

Drug and Supplement Use and Your Health

19

The Whole Truth About Drugs

Activity A

Chapter 19

Name _____

Date _____ Period_____

Following are 19 sets of statements about drugs. Each set contains three statements, which will either be all correct or all incorrect. For each of the 19 sets of statements, circle "Yes" in the box on the right if all three statements are correct and "No" if all three statements are incorrect. For each "No," use the far-right column to show changes needed in the underlined words to make each statement true. Study the example given in #1.

1.	a. Drugs are substances, <u>including</u> foods, that change the ways the mind or body functions.	**Yes** or **(No)**	other than
	b. Medicines are drugs used to <u>prevent</u> ailments or improve disabling conditions.		treat
	c. Ergogenic aids are substances intended to enhance <u>physical appearance</u>.		strength and endurance
2.	a. Prescription drugs are sold legally <u>without</u> an order from a doctor.	**Yes** or **No**	
	b. Over-the-counter drugs can be obtained <u>only with</u> an order from a doctor.		
	c. Illegal drugs are <u>lawful</u> to buy or use.		
3.	a. The chemical name of a drug describes the drug's <u>chemical</u> composition.	**Yes** or **No**	
	b. The <u>generic</u> name is the officially accepted name of a drug.		
	c. The <u>brand or trade</u> name is the name used by the manufacturer to promote a drug product.		
4.	a. A <u>food-drug interaction</u> happens when drugs, supplements, and foods have physical and chemical effects on one another.	**Yes** or **No**	
	b. A drug's <u>side effect</u> is a reaction that differs from its desired effect.		
	c. <u>Tolerance</u> is the ability of the mind and body to become less responsive to a drug.		

(Continued)

5.	a. The definition of drug <u>abuse</u> is using a substance other than food or water to change the way the body or mind functions.	**Yes or No**	
	b. Drug misuse occurs when medicine is <u>intentionally</u> used in a way that proves harmful.		
	c. Drug abuse occurs when drugs are <u>unintentionally</u> used for nonmedical reasons that can put a person's health at risk.		
6.	a. An addiction is a <u>social</u> dependence on a drug.	**Yes or No**	
	b. Withdrawal happens when a person <u>starts</u> taking an addictive drug.		
	c. Tolerance is the ability of the mind and body to become <u>more</u> responsive to a drug.		
7.	a. <u>Psychoactive</u> drugs affect the central nervous system.	**Yes or No**	
	b. Stimulants <u>speed up</u> the nervous system.		
	c. Depressants <u>decrease</u> the activity of the central nervous system.		
8.	a. Caffeine is a <u>mild</u> stimulant drug.	**Yes or No**	
	b. <u>Amphetamines</u> are commonly abused stimulants.		
	c. <u>Cocaine</u> affects the brain within seconds after use.		
9.	a. Secondhand smoke <u>does not</u> contain cancer-causing compounds.	**Yes or No**	
	b. Smokeless tobacco contains <u>tar</u>, making it addictive and harmful to health.		
	c. Snuff is an example of <u>smoked</u> tobacco.		
10.	a. Alcohol <u>is not</u> a drug.	**Yes or No**	
	b. Alcohol can be absorbed through the walls of the <u>small intestine</u>, unlike carbohydrates, fats, and proteins.		
	c. The effects of alcohol consumption on the body are relatively <u>slow</u>.		
11.	a. Alcohol causes the body to <u>retain</u> water.	**Yes or No**	
	b. Alcohol <u>speeds up</u> reaction times.		
	c. Alcohol <u>increases</u> body coordination.		

(Continued)

12.	a. Tranquilizers are sometimes prescribed for people who are feeling overly <u>anxious</u>.	**Yes or No**	
	b. Barbiturates are sometimes prescribed for people who have difficulty <u>sleeping</u>.		
	c. Inhalants have mind-numbing effects and <u>are not</u> prescribed.		
13.	a. Most <u>narcotics</u> are made from the opium poppy.	**Yes or No**	
	b. Codeine and morphine are <u>opiates</u>.		
	c. Heroin is the <u>most</u> addictive narcotic known today.		
14.	a. Marijuana <u>is not</u> a hallucinogen.	**Yes or No**	
	b. <u>LSD</u> is the main mood-altering ingredient in marijuana.		
	c. Marijuana cigarettes release <u>the same amount of</u> carbon monoxide into the lungs as tobacco cigarettes.		
15.	a. Ecstasy is known as a "<u>club drug</u>."	**Yes or No**	
	b. Ecstasy is both a <u>stimulant</u> and a hallucinogen.		
	c. Ecstasy is dangerously harmful to the <u>brain</u>.		
16.	a. LSD and PCP are both <u>hallucinogens</u>.	**Yes or No**	
	b. LSD and PCP are made in <u>illegal</u> labs.		
	c. LSD and PCP users often engage in <u>dangerous</u> behaviors.		
17.	a. Designer drugs are created in <u>legal</u> labs.	**Yes or No**	
	b. Designer drugs are much <u>weaker</u> than the drugs they imitate.		
	c. Designer drugs are <u>usually</u> tested for contaminants.		
18.	a. Anabolic steroids are <u>natural</u> hormones used to build muscles.	**Yes or No**	
	b. Anabolic steroids are a version of the hormone <u>estrogen</u>.		
	c. Using anabolic steroids can <u>boost</u> fertility.		
19.	a. Dietary supplements <u>must be</u> approved by the FDA.	**Yes or No**	
	b. Most supplements have <u>much</u> research to back up their advertising claims.		
	c. Dietary supplements and ergogenic aids <u>are not</u> the same thing.		

Psychoactive Drugs

Name _____

Date _____ Period_____

Complete the following chart to organize important facts about psychoactive drugs.

Drug	Stimulant, depressant, or hallucinogen	Sources or uses	Physical effects	Related diseases	Recommendations
caffeine					
amphetamines					
cocaine					
nicotine					
alcohol					
barbiturates					
tranquilizers					
inhalants					
narcotics					
marijuana					
Ecstasy					
LSD/PCP					

Common-Sense Comebacks

Many drug abusers started using and misusing drugs at the urgings of other people. Some people find it hard to turn down an invitation, even when it goes against common knowledge and good sense. Use facts from the chapter to write a good "comeback" or response for each of the invitations below.

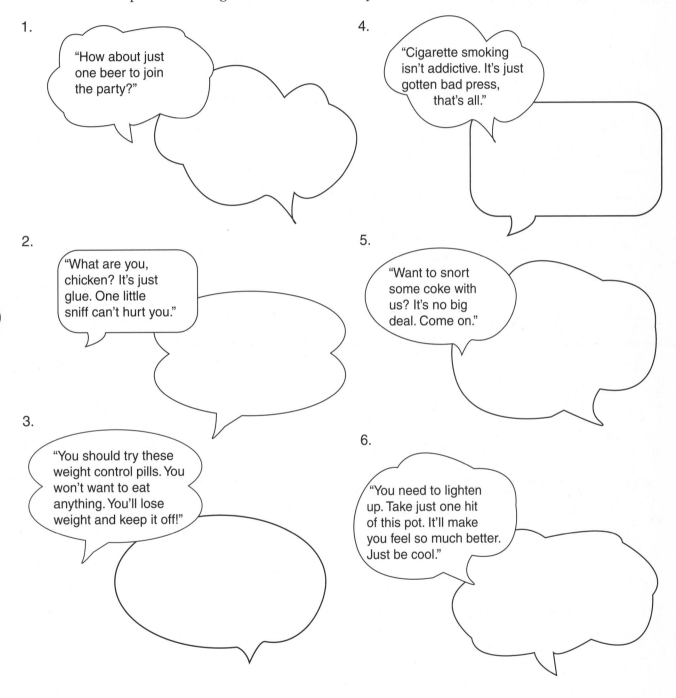

1.

"How about just one beer to join the party?"

4.

"Cigarette smoking isn't addictive. It's just gotten bad press, that's all."

2.

"What are you, chicken? It's just glue. One little sniff can't hurt you."

5.

"Want to snort some coke with us? It's no big deal. Come on."

3.

"You should try these weight control pills. You won't want to eat anything. You'll lose weight and keep it off!"

6.

"You need to lighten up. Take just one hit of this pot. It'll make you feel so much better. Just be cool."

What Do You Think?

Name _____

Date _____ Period_____

For each of the following statements about drug use, put a check in the column—Agree, Unsure, or Disagree—that best reflects your views. Then answer the questions at the bottom of the page and explain your answers.

Agree   Unsure   Disagree

_____ _____ _____   1. It is wrong to use any illegal drug.

_____ _____ _____   2. It is all right to use another person's prescription medicine if he or she gives it to you.

_____ _____ _____   3. The legal age for buying tobacco products should be lowered.

_____ _____ _____   4. A person convicted of drinking and driving should have his or her license revoked.

_____ _____ _____   5. Smoking should be banned in all public places.

_____ _____ _____   6. It is all right to use illegal drugs if no one finds out about it.

_____ _____ _____   7. I wish alcohol were illegal for everyone.

_____ _____ _____   8. Athletes should not be allowed to use anabolic steroids—it gives them an unfair advantage.

_____ _____ _____   9. All drugs should be legal.

_____ _____ _____ 10. People who sell drugs to children should be put in jail.

_____ _____ _____ 11. The drinking age should be lowered.

_____ _____ _____ 12. People who furnish alcohol or cigarettes to minors should be fined or arrested.

_____ _____ _____ 13. Athletes should be allowed to use anabolic steroids if they want—it's their bodies.

_____ _____ _____ 14. Penalties for driving while drinking should be less harsh.

_____ _____ _____ 15. People should stop trying to ban smoking in public.

16. If someone who agreed with statement number _____ wanted to be my friend, I would have to think twice. Explain. _____

_____

_____

17. If someone I was dating disagreed with statement number _____, I would have to reconsider the relationship. Explain. _____

_____

_____

18. Final comments on drug use and abuse: _____

_____

_____

Backtrack
Through Chapter 19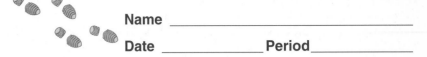

Activity E

Chapter 19

Name _____

Date _____ Period_____

Provide complete answers to the following questions and statements about drug use and abuse.

Recall the Facts

- -

1. Why are doctors the only people who can write drug prescriptions? _____

   _____

2. Is a brand-name drug better than the same drug in generic form? Why or why not? _____

   _____

3. How do prices of brand-name drugs compare with those of generic drugs? _____

   _____

4. List five factors that affect the way the body uses the chemicals from drugs. _____

   _____

5. What is the difference between drug misuse and drug abuse? _____

   _____

6. What are the three main types of psychoactive drugs? _____

   _____

7. Name seven symptoms of drug withdrawal. _____

   _____

8. Of the drugs described in the chapter, which one kills the most people? _____

9. By how many minutes is a person's life shortened with each cigarette smoked? _____

10. Smokers need more vitamin C than nonsmokers. How much extra vitamin C do smokers need per day, and why? _____

    _____

11. If a person is trying to quit smoking, is smokeless tobacco a good substitute? Why or why not?

    _____

12. Why are designer drugs especially dangerous? _____

    _____

13. Name three community resources that can help alcoholics and their families. _____

    _____

(Continued)

Interpret Implications

14. What are the symptoms of caffeine withdrawal and how can they be minimized? _____
   _____
   _____

15. Why have amphetamines been found largely ineffective for weight control? _____
   _____
   _____

16. Explain the effects of tar that collects in the lungs of smokers. _____
   _____
   _____

17. Explain why many alcoholics find it difficult to get help. _____
   _____

18. Explain why the use of anabolic steroids can be dangerous. _____
   _____
   _____

Apply & Practice

19. List five tips for consumers buying OTC drug products. _____
   _____
   _____
   _____

20. Write a short paragraph describing how you would feel and what you would do if you knew
   someone close to you was planning to use ergogenic aids. _____
   _____
   _____

21. Write a short paragraph describing how you would feel and what you would do if you knew
   someone close to you was misusing or abusing drugs.
   _____
   _____
   _____
   _____

Keeping Food Safe

20

The Contaminators

Activity A

Chapter 20

Name _____

Date _____ Period_____

Food contaminants, or "contaminators," are undesirable substances that may unintentionally get into food. In order to protect the food supply from the harmful effects of contaminants, you must first learn to identify these types of undesirable substances. Food contaminants do not carry ID cards, but if they did, perhaps they would look something like these. Fill in the blank in each ID card to identify types of food contaminants.

ID Contaminator 1

I am a single-celled microorganism. I live in soil, water, and bodies of plants and animals. I am _____.

ID Contaminator 2

I am an organism that lives off another organism called a *host*. I am a _____.

ID Contaminator 3

I am an agent that causes diseases. I am the smallest type of life form. I am a _____.

ID Contaminator 4

I am particles left behind after poisons such as insect repellant or weed killer are sprayed on plants. I am _____.

ID Contaminator 5

I am chemical substances that are released into the air by an industrial plant. I make my way into the food supply. I am _____.

ID Contaminator 6

In addition to being known as a poison, I am also known as a _____.

ID Contaminator 7

I may be a bacterium, parasite, virus, or fungus. We are all known as _____.

ID Contaminator 8

I am a mold. I am a type of _____.

ID Contaminator 9

I am a yeast. I am a type of _____.

ID Contaminator 10

I am a single-celled animal. I am a parasite. I cause foodborne illness. I am _____.

Safe Shopping List

Activity B

Chapter 20

Name _____

Date _____ Period_____

Read the following food shopping scenarios. Use ideas from the scenarios to help you develop a list of tips for safe food shopping. Record your list of tips in the space provided.

Scenario 1:

A foul odor greeted Jeremy in the produce section at Super Market. He had trouble finding fresh broccoli that looked good. Instead, Jeremy went to the frozen foods case to get frozen broccoli. There he found some broccoli spears, but all the packages were covered with frost! As a last resort, Jeremy decided to serve string beans instead of broccoli and headed for the canned goods aisle.

Scenario 2:

Donnie stopped at Buy Mart to pick up some deli foods for the family picnic. His sister had said the store appeared sloppy, but it was a convenient place to stop on the way to the lake. He noticed some of the cartons of potato salad had expired dates and others had no labels. A few had loosened lids or were stacked well above the level of cold air in the case. Donnie was careful to select only those with current dates and tightly closed lids. He also chose cartons that were stored deep down in the case.

Scenario 3:

Jan heard about the weekend specials at the Corner Grocery. When she reached the back of the store, she started having second thoughts. The meat case was stained with meat drippings. She did not see the cuts she needed in the meat case, but no one was on duty to help her. Finally, she picked a package of cut-up chicken and went to the checkout. Only after she got home did she realize the chicken had leaked all over her lettuce. What a mess!

Safe Shopping

_____

_____

_____

_____

_____

_____

_____

_____

_____

_____

_____

_____

_____

_____

_____

_____

_____

_____

Food at Home and on the Go

Read the following statements about food handling practices at home and away from home. If the statement is true, write the word *true* in the blank. If the statement is false, change the underlined word(s) to make the statement true. Write the correct word(s) in the blank.

_____ 1. Store eggs on the shelf located <u>on the door</u> of the refrigerator.

_____ 2. When you get home from the store, put away <u>perishable</u> foods first.

_____ 3. Keep the refrigerator at a temperature of <u>0</u>°F.

_____ 4. Keep a <u>meat</u> thermometer in your freezer to ensure a safe temperature.

_____ 5. Store dry beans in <u>the refrigerator</u>.

_____ 6. Chill cooked foods <u>quickly</u> to minimize growth of bacteria.

_____ 7. <u>Air circulation</u> helps foods chill more quickly.

_____ 8. Most leftovers will keep safely in the refrigerator for <u>three to four weeks</u>.

_____ 9. <u>Wax paper</u> and plastic wrap are suitable disposable food covers.

_____ 10. The sink base cabinet <u>is</u> a good place to store potatoes and onions.

_____ 11. Wash hands with soap and warm water for <u>20</u> seconds before handling food.

_____ 12. You <u>do</u> need to wash your hands after each time you cough or sneeze.

_____ 13. Wear gloves in the kitchen when you have a <u>cold</u>.

_____ 14. A <u>plastic</u> cutting board is easier to clean than a wooden one.

_____ 15. <u>Bacteria</u> can grow on the blade of a can opener if it is not kept clean.

_____ 16. <u>Damp</u> dishcloths and sponges are breeding grounds for bacteria.

_____ 17. Bacteria grow <u>least</u> rapidly at temperatures between 40°F and 140°F.

_____ 18. Limit time foods are held at room temperature to no more than <u>four</u> hours.

_____ 19. Refrigerate leftovers <u>only after cooling to room temperature</u>.

_____ 20. The safest place to thaw foods is <u>on the kitchen counter</u>.

_____ 21. It is a good idea to <u>taste</u> meat before serving to be sure it is completely done.

_____ 22. Undercooked eggs may contain <u>*E. coli*</u> bacteria.

_____ 23. Microwave ovens tend to cook foods <u>less</u> evenly than regular ovens.

_____ 24. Pack food to go in an <u>insulated</u> bag or cooler.

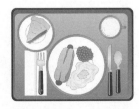

Out of the Danger Zone

Use the thermometer diagram below to answer questions about the temperature danger zone.

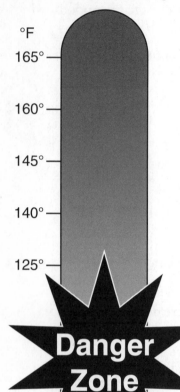

°F

165° —

160° —

145° —

140° —

125° —

Danger Zone

60° —

40° —

0° —

Part 1

Put an A, B, and C next to the temperatures on the thermometer diagram for each of the following:

A. optimum holding temperature for cooked foods

B. optimum temperature for refrigerator storage of foods

C. optimum temperature for freezer storage of foods

Part 2

Write "DZ" in the space before each food below that is in the "Danger Zone." (Note: All temperatures are Fahrenheit.)

_____ A. Egg salad sandwiches in a hiker's backpack on a 30°F day

_____ B. Chicken and other food purchases in a parked car on an 80°F day

_____ C. Hamburger stored in an insulated cooler at 60°F

_____ D. Eggs on the refrigerator door shelf at 50°F

_____ E. Fish nuggets held on a buffet at 145°F

_____ F. Casserole in a 0°F freezer

_____ G. Stuffed turkey left on the table at room temperature

_____ H. Leftover deviled eggs in a 42°F refrigerator

_____ I. Chocolate pudding in 39°F refrigerator

_____ J. Fried chicken at a picnic on a 92°F day

_____ K. Cooked rice on the kitchen counter

_____ L. Lamb chops in a freezer at -5°F

Food Safety Is No Accident

Name _____

Date _____ Period_____

Choose the best response. Write the letter in the space provided.

_____ 1. A system used to protect the food supply by identifying steps at which food products may be at risk of contamination is _____.
   A. Hazard Analysis Critical Control Point (HACCP)
   B. Hazard Identification Critical Contamination Point (HICCP)
   C. Hazard Protection Contamination Control Point (HPCCP)
   D. Hazard Risk Control Contamination Point (HRCCP)

_____ 2. Keeping clean everything that comes in contact with food to help prevent disease is called _____.
   A. additive
   B. control point
   C. cross-contamination
   D. sanitation

_____ 3. Personal practices, such as hand washing, that promote safe foods and good health are called _____.
   A. hygiene
   B. management
   C. planning
   D. preparation

_____ 4. The transfer of harmful bacteria from one food to another due to unsafe food preparation or storage practices is called _____.
   A. cross-contamination
   B. environmental contaminant
   C. foodborne illness
   D. food poisoning

_____ 5. The "Danger Zone" in which food bacteria are likely to thrive is between _____.
   A. 20°C–120°C
   B. 20°F–120°F
   C. 40°C–140°C
   D. 40°F–140°F

_____ 6. People who work with food and have cuts on their hands should _____.
   A. go to the doctor
   B. not work with food
   C. wash in boiling hot water
   D. wear gloves

_____ 7. To reduce the risk of spreading food bacteria while working with meats, use tools and cutting boards that _____.
   A. are dried with cloth towels
   B. are easy to clean
   C. have porous surfaces
   D. are made of wood

_____ 8. Reactions to illness-causing bacteria _____.
   A. vary from one person to another
   B. are affected by one's genetic makeup
   C. are affected by one's state of health
   D. All the above.

_____ 9. The group of people listed below at lowest risk for foodborne illness is _____.
   A. adolescents
   B. alcoholics
   C. elderly people
   D. pregnant females

(Continued)

_____ 10. The most common symptoms of foodborne illness are _____.
   A. vomiting, skin rash, and headache
   B. chills, diarrhea, and headache
   C. dizziness, vomiting, and fatigue
   D. vomiting, diarrhea, and stomach cramps

_____ 11. Symptoms of most foodborne illness _____.
   A. appear within a few hours and last less than one day
   B. appear within a day or two and last a few days
   C. appear within a week or two and last a few days
   D. appear within 30 days and last a few weeks

_____ 12. When you are in doubt about the safety of a food, _____.
   A. take a small bite to see if it has an off taste
   B. check to see if it smells spoiled
   C. bring it to a boil to kill the bacteria
   D. None of the above.

_____ 13. For mild symptoms of foodborne illness, _____.
   A. call the doctor immediately
   B. drink lots of fluids and rest
   C. eat lots of fiber and rest
   D. take aspirin and drink lots of fluids

_____ 14. Symptoms of severe foodborne illness are _____.
   A. fever, blood in stools, dehydration, and dizziness
   B. cramps, vomiting, diarrhea, and fever
   C. dizziness, headache, fever, and chills
   D. diarrhea, abdominal pain, and headache

_____ 15. Double vision, inability to swallow, and difficulty speaking are symptoms of _____.
   A. *E. coli* poisoning
   B. toxicity
   C. botulism
   D. trichinosis

_____ 16. You should file a report of a foodborne illness if the food _____.
   A. came from a public source
   B. was served to a large number of people
   C. was a commercial product
   D. All the above.

_____ 17. Which of the following is the correct sequence for the food supply chain?
   A. Food consumers, food producers, food processors, and government agencies.
   B. Food processors, food producers, consumers, and government agencies.
   C. Food producers, food processors, government agencies, and consumers.
   D. Farmers, food consumers, food processors, and government agencies.

_____ 18. Safe use of pesticides is a responsibility of _____.
   A. food processors
   B. food producers
   C. consumers
   D. All the above.

_____ 19. The government agency that regulates food advertising is _____.
   A. USDA
   B. FTC
   C. EPA
   D. FDA

_____ 20. The government agency that inspects fish products is the _____.
   A. FSIS
   B. EPA
   C. USDA
   D. NMFS

Backtrack
Through Chapter 20

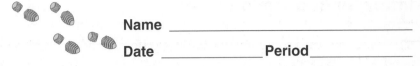

Activity F

Chapter 20

Name _____

Date _____ Period_____

Provide complete answers to the following questions and statements about food safety.

Recall the Facts

1. Why do many cases of foodborne illness go unreported? _____
   _____

2. What is the chief cause of foodborne illness in the United States? _____

3. List five types of bacteria that can cause foodborne illnesses._____
   _____

4. What two viruses may be contracted from contaminated raw or undercooked shellfish? _____
   _____

5. List five main steps for outwitting food contaminators._____
   _____
   _____

6. How can food processors help ensure a safe food supply? _____
   _____
   _____

7. What foods are monitored by the USDA and FSIS? _____

8. What foods are monitored by the FDA? _____

9. Who checks food handling in local grocery stores and food service operations? _____

10. What are a consumer's responsibilities with regard to food safety? _____
    _____
    _____

(Continued)

Interpret Implications

11. Can a person avoid foodborne illness completely by avoiding foods that look, smell, and taste bad? Why? _____

    _____

12. Explain why attention to time and temperature is necessary for keeping food safe._____

    _____

13. Why should moldy foods be discarded?_____

    _____

14. If you have many errands, why should you save food shopping for last? _____

    _____

15. List two precautions you should take when cooking marinated meats. _____

    _____

    _____

16. Why are children at greater risk of foodborne illness than adults? _____

    _____

17. Why would you want to keep food you suspect has made you ill? _____

    _____

Apply & Practice

18. How can you protect yourself from pesticide residues?_____

    _____

    _____

    _____

19. How can you protect yourself from environmental contaminants found in fish? _____

    _____

20. What personal hygiene habits have you violated or seen violated by others when working with food?

    _____

    _____

    _____

21

A Meal Manager in the Making

Activity A

Chapter 21

Name _____

Date _____ Period_____

Meg writes in her diary some of her experiences in meal planning and preparation. Identify the advantage of meal planning that is not being realized in each of Meg's entries. Select from the following list: *appeal, nutrition, economy,* and *saving time and effort*. List tips that would have prevented Meg's problems each day and helped her become a better meal manager.

Sept. 2—Our first dinner in the apartment was no picnic! It took all afternoon to cook and most of the evening to clean up the kitchen. I couldn't find anything in that kitchen. I had to stop twice and run down to the convenience store for ingredients I needed. That stuffing recipe had the longest list of ingredients I've ever seen. What are shallots, anyway? I thought the turkey would never get done! I've learned my lesson!

1. Advantage Missing: _____

2. Tips: _____

_____

Sept. 4—Sorry, Diary, but I've been too busy to write. We're having turkey again tonight. Boy, am I tired of turkey sandwiches on white bread. I know we can't afford to waste the turkey, so maybe we can bear it just one more night. I'll boil some potatoes to go with it, and we can have a bowl of vanilla ice cream.

3. Advantage Missing: _____

4. Tips: _____

_____

Sept. 5—Well, it's four for dinner again tonight. Diane won't be here, but Beth is bringing home a friend. The catch is she's a vegetarian—I guess that rules out turkey sandwiches. Maybe I could just fix sandwiches for the rest of us and warm up some canned vegetables for Beth's friend. That sounds like a plan.

5. Advantage Missing: _____

6. Tips: _____

_____

Sept. 6—Since the turkey's finally gone, I stopped by the grocery store today to shop for tonight's dinner. Luckily, I had all the money for this month's food budget with me. I was so hungry! I picked up a few snack items. I couldn't resist the fresh asparagus, even though it was out of season and very expensive. I found four of the best-looking Porterhouse steaks. I thought we could grill outside to keep from heating the apartment. The meal was great. Everyone loved it. The only problem now is how we are going to eat for the rest of the month.

7. Advantage Missing: _____

8. Tips: _____

_____

Menu Makeovers

Each menu below lacks variety in one of the following ways: flavor, color, texture, shape and size, or temperature. For each menu, determine which type of variety is most lacking and write it in the blank under the arrow. Use the block on the right to do a menu makeover that will improve variety.

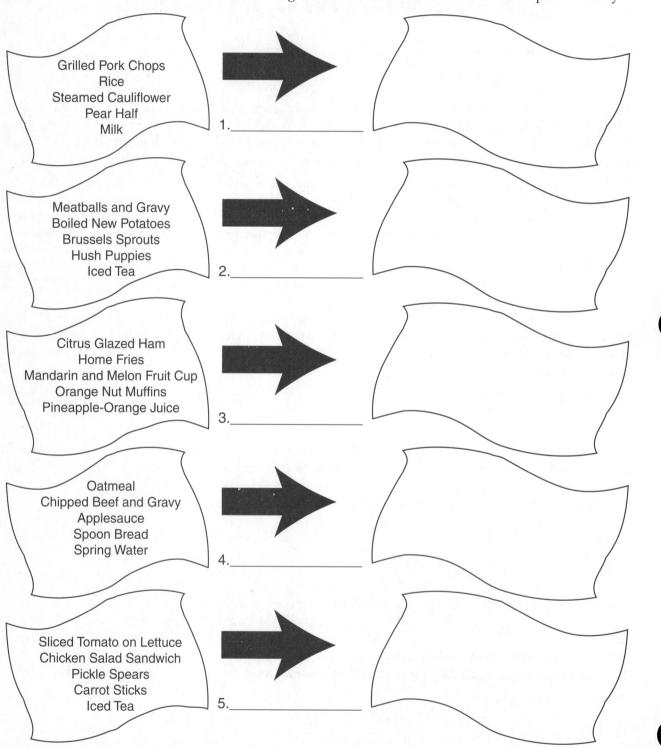

Grilled Pork Chops
Rice
Steamed Cauliflower
Pear Half
Milk

1._____

Meatballs and Gravy
Boiled New Potatoes
Brussels Sprouts
Hush Puppies
Iced Tea

2._____

Citrus Glazed Ham
Home Fries
Mandarin and Melon Fruit Cup
Orange Nut Muffins
Pineapple-Orange Juice

3._____

Oatmeal
Chipped Beef and Gravy
Applesauce
Spoon Bread
Spring Water

4._____

Sliced Tomato on Lettuce
Chicken Salad Sandwich
Pickle Spears
Carrot Sticks
Iced Tea

5._____

Three Squares Plus

Name _____

Date _____ Period_____

A typical way of meeting nutritional needs is to plan three square meals a day plus a nutritious snack. Use the squares provided to plan a nutritious menu for one day using foods you enjoy. Keep in mind lunch and dinner should each supply one-third of your daily nutritional needs. Breakfast should furnish one-fourth of your needs and a snack should provide the rest. Then answer the question at the bottom of the page.

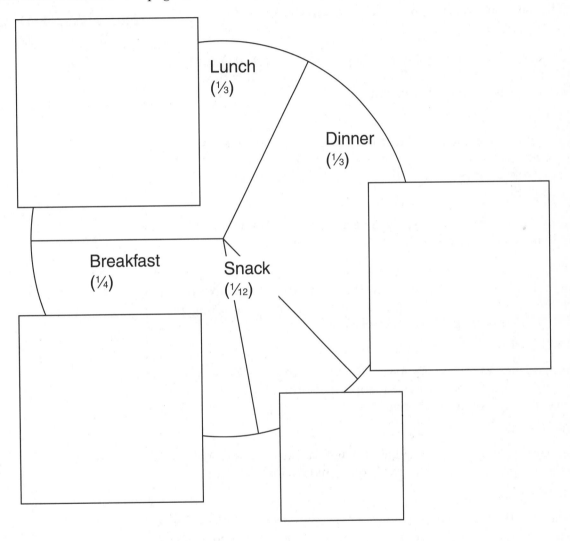

Must everyone follow the "three squares plus" eating pattern each day in order to be healthy? Explain.

_____

_____

_____

Budgeting Dilemmas

Name _____

Date _____ **Period**_____

Pretend you have budgeted $50 a month for food. This includes eating out and buying any grocery items not purchased by your family. Use your food money wisely. Read each of the following situations and decide what to do. Write your decision about each item before reading any further. Use the notepad on the right to calculate your spending. Then answer the questions about your spending.

1. January 4: A friend invites you to the mall. You are hungry, and Chinese food looks good. The meal you like costs $4.75.

   You decide: _____

2. January 7: You want to start eating yogurt at breakfast. Your family doesn't eat yogurt, so you'll have to buy it. At the grocery store, yogurt costs $3.25 for five containers.

   You decide: _____

3. January 9: At school, you like to buy juice from the vending machine at lunch each day. One carton of juice costs 55 cents. There are 19 school days this month.

   You decide: _____

4. January 11: When your family is visiting a museum, you want lemonade ($2.00) and nachos ($2.50) from the snack bar.

   You decide: _____

5. January 17: You and a date go to a movie. It is your turn to buy refreshments. Your date suggests you each get a medium popcorn and large soft drink. The total price is $9.

   You decide: _____

6. January 18: You're buying snacks for a party at your house. You can't decide whether to serve a fruit salad or banana splits. In either case, the ingredients cost about $8.

   You decide: _____

7. January 19: You are studying for a test with a friend. Your friend wants to have a pizza delivered. Each of you would pay half (about $7.50).

   You decide: _____

8. January 21: Your mom's birthday is next week. You want to surprise her with a cake. You could make it yourself (ingredients total about $7) or order it specially made from the store bakery ($15).

   You decide: _____

9. January 26: You think about asking a date to dinner. At the restaurant you have chosen, you expect dinner and tip to cost at least $20.

   You decide: _____

10. January 31: On your class field trip, lunch is in the Capitol building restaurant. You can eat: a salad ($2.99); soup and salad, ($3.50); or a hamburger and fries ($4.99).

    You decide: _____

Budget Notebook

| January | $50 |

(Continued)

11. At the end of the month, how much had you spent on food? _____

12. How did this compare to the $50 you had budgeted? _____
_____

13. Were there any purchases you made that were poor decisions? Why? _____
_____
_____

14. What other purchases would you have made if you had budgeted more money for food? _____
_____

15. How do the decisions in this activity compare to food decisions you must make in your life?
Explain. _____
_____
_____
_____
_____
_____

16. How might setting a food budget help you control your food spending? Explain. _____
_____
_____
_____

Eating Out and About

Name _____

Date _____ Period_____

Eating meals away from home is a challenge for meal managers today. Prepare a list of tips for nutritional eating when you are "out and about" and record tips in the spaces provided. Prepare a menu for a nutritious meal or snack in each category.

Tips for Packing Lunches

Tips for Takeout

Menu

Menu

Menu

Menu

Tips for Snacking from Vending Machines

Tips for Buffet Dinner

Backtrack
Through Chapter 21

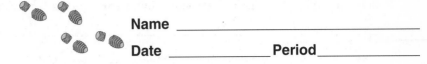

Activity F

Chapter 21

Name _____

Date _____ Period _____

Provide complete answers to the following questions and statements about meal management.

Recall the Facts

1. Name four advantages of planning meals. _____

   _____

2. Name five ways you can add variety to make meals more enjoyable. _____

   _____

3. What resources can meal managers use to help meet nutritional needs? _____

   _____

4. Give three examples of special needs that may need to be addressed during meal planning. ____

   _____

   _____

5. Following the Dietary Guidelines for Americans will help you control what in your diet? _____

   _____

   _____

6. What is a healthy cooking method? _____

   _____

7. What is a budget? _____

   _____

8. Name five examples of time-saving appliances. _____

   _____

9. What are convenience foods? _____

   _____

10. Name three items you can order in fast-food restaurants to substitute for less-nutritious selections.

    _____

Interpret Implications

11. Explain two reasons for serving a variety of foods. _____

    _____

(Continued)

12. When preparing a healthy meal, what factors must you consider? Give an example of each. _____

_____

_____

_____

13. List three tips to keep in mind when preparing a food budget. _____

_____

_____

14. Name two tools you would store near each of the following locations:

 A. sink _____

 B. range _____

 C. refrigerator _____

 D. table _____

15. What are three advantages of convenience foods? _____

_____

16. What are two disadvantages of convenience foods? _____

_____

17. Name an advantage of packed lunches for eating away from home. _____

_____

Apply & Practice

- -

18. List two goals you have related to meal management. List resources that can help you reach each goal.

_____

_____

19. Compare your nutritional needs with those of a family member with different nutritional needs. How does your family manage meals to accommodate these different needs? _____

_____

_____

20. List five relatively high-cost foods. For each, list a replacement food from the same food group that is relatively low in cost. _____

_____

_____

Where to Shop?

Activity A

Chapter 22

Name _____

Date _____ Period_____

Match the terms with their identifying phrases.

A. convenience store

B. cooperative

C. farmers' market

D. outlet store

E. roadside stand

F. specialty store

G. supermarket

H. warehouse store

_____ 1. Group of produce stands offered by a group of farmers, often in a city location.

_____ 2. Store that sells many food items in large containers and multiunit packages.

_____ 3. Grocery store that offers many products and services in addition to food.

_____ 4. Store that sells products made by one food manufacturer.

_____ 5. Store that stays open around the clock so people can stop in and quickly pick up a few items.

_____ 6. Food store that is owned and operated by members who can buy food there at a discount.

_____ 7. Produce stand offered by an individual farmer during growing season.

In the section below, read the shopper's main concern. For each item, write in the type of store the shopper could choose to best satisfy this concern.

_____ 8. Trudy does not have a car and prefers to shop for everything she needs by going online.

_____ 9. Tom is at home late one evening and realizes he is out of bread. He wants to just run in, buy the bread, and get home to make his sandwich.

_____ 10. Amelia wants to shop somewhere that isn't crowded. In fact, she would like a place that is not open to the public.

_____ 11. Carl likes a large selection. He also prefers to have his prescriptions filled while he is shopping.

_____ 12. Armando needs the freshest fruit for a recipe. He lives in the city and doesn't have time to travel far.

_____ 13. Lisa and her husband have seven children. They like to buy frozen foods, peanut butter, and other items in large quantities. This helps them save money.

_____ 14. Keisha prefers to get her meat directly from a butcher because the quality of meat is better.

_____ 15. Kimberly likes to buy a certain brand of bread products. She doesn't mind if the bread is somewhat misshapen—if the price is right.

What Influences Shopping Decisions?

Activity B

Chapter 22

Name _____

Date _____ Period_____

Interview the person in your home who does most of the food shopping for your family. If possible, conduct the interview just after a trip to the store. Record responses below, and share your findings with the class.

Section I. Advertising as an Influence

1. Think of a specific product you have bought recently. List the item here: _____

   A. Have you seen any advertising on this product? _____

   B. If so, what medium of advertising was used? _____

   C. Do you think the ad had any influence on your decision to buy the product? _____

   D. What type of impression, if any, did the ad make on you? _____

   _____

   E. Did the ad focus on facts about the product? Explain. _____

   _____

   F. Did the ad try to appeal to your basic needs or desires? Did it claim or imply the product could improve your life in some way? Explain. _____

   _____

Section 2. Form of Food as an Influence

2. Which form of each of the following products do you purchase most often? For each product, circle your response and explain your choice.

   A. Bread: Plain white bread   Enriched white bread   Whole-grain bread

   Reason: _____

   B. Green beans: Fresh   Canned   Frozen

   Reason: _____

   C. Chicken: Whole fresh   Cut fresh   Frozen breasts   Cooked, ready-to-eat

   Reason: _____

   D. Butter/margarine: Butter   Regular margarine   Fortified margarine

   Reason: _____

Section 3. Health as an Influence

3. Do you generally read the ingredient lists and nutritional information on food labels? Why or why not?

   _____

4. What food additives, if any, do you try to avoid or minimize in your food purchases? _____

   _____

(Continued)

5. Do you buy organic foods? Why or why not? _____

_____

6. Do you wash fruits and vegetables before using? Why or why not? _____

_____

Section 4. Price as an Influence

7. Do you generally compare prices and quality of similar products before choosing what to buy? Why or why not?

_____

_____

8. Do you use unit pricing information? Why or why not? _____

_____

9. Which do you tend to buy most often—national brands, store brands, or generic products? Explain. _____

_____

10. Do you use a shopping list? _____
    A. Is your list organized by category, such as meats, dairy products, and frozen foods? _____
    B. Do you plan menus before you determine what items to put on the list? _____
    C. Do you consult recipes as needed for lists of ingredients to be purchased? _____
    D. Do you keep a running list of items needed as you run out of things during the week? ____
    E. Do you review advertised specials to aid in making your list? _____
    F. Do you often use coupons when shopping for food items? _____

11. Do you tend to purchase items on impulse? _____
    A. Do you avoid shopping when you are hungry or tired? _____
    B. Do you try to select foods that are in season? _____
    C. Do you tend to be drawn to store displays of items not on your shopping list? _____

Deciphering Food Claims

Name _____

Date _____ Period_____

The chart below lists four types of food claims found on food labels. For each claim, provide a definition, an example from the text, and your own example. You may use information found on pages 530 to 533 of the text.

Claim type	Definition	Text example	Student example			
			Food	**Brand**	**Claim**	**What it means**
Nutrient content claims						
Health claims						
Qualified health claims						
Structure and function claims						

Food Shopping in the Know

Name _____

Date _____ Period_____

The chart below has a list of 17 terms related to food shopping. For each term, write the definition in the middle column. Then select the example from the list that best exemplifies the term. Write the letter code—a through q—for the example in the right-hand column.

Term	Definition	Example
1. consumer		
2. food processing		
3. food irradiation		
4. food additive		
5. generally recognized as safe list		
6. organic foods		
7. comparison shopping		
8. unit price		
9. national brand		
10. store brand		
11. generic product		

(Continued)

12. allergen labeling		
13. country-of-origin label		
14. claims labeling		
15. impulse buying		
16. serving size		
17. right to redress		

Examples:

A.   An egg carton has a green and white symbol with two leaf-shapes in the center.

B.   The shelf tag in the canned soup section reads "8 cents per ounce."

C.   The farmer uses a hoe to eliminate weeds and a natural solution to eliminate pests in his crops.

D.   The manufacturer is required to list peanuts and wheat on the ingredients list.

E.   The shopper takes time to check the costs of fresh, canned, and frozen peaches before deciding which to buy.

F.   The shopper buys the brand of popcorn he saw advertised on TV.

G.   Sugar and salt are both on the GRAS list.

H.   Shelley eats ½ cup of ice cream at a time, while Sherman eats a full cup.

I.   Harriet buys soups in the plain cans because they are fine for everyday dishes.

J.   The COOL label on the avocadoes reads "Mexico."

K.   The label lists two ingredients acting as preservatives in the jar of spaghetti sauce.

L.   The label on the milk carton reads "pasteurized."

M.   Laura buys the Bigmart cereals because they are cheaper.

N.   As he waits in line to check out, Calvin grabs a few items off a nearby shelf and adds them to his basket.

O.   The consumer reports her problem with the faulty refrigerator and the uncooperative company to the Better Business Bureau.

P.   The food label reads: "Diets rich in sodium may reduce the risk of high blood pressure."

Q.   You and anyone else who buys and uses products and services.

Savvy Shopper or Careless Consumer?

Activity E

Chapter 22

Name _____

Date _____ Period _____

A savvy shopper is knowledgeable about fitness products and services and uses available information to make informed choices. A careless consumer, on the other hand, does not plan ahead, ask questions, or compare prices and quality. Read the shopping scenarios below. In the blanks on the left, write *SS* if the text describes a savvy shopper and *CC* for each illustration of a careless consumer. Use the space beneath each scenario to identify the practice that was either savvy or careless.

_____ 1. Darrin decided to purchase his hiking boots on the Internet. It would be much easier than fighting crowds at the local mall. He was pretty sure he knew what size to get. He wasn't too concerned by the online store's policy of no refunds and no exchanges.

Practice: _____

_____ 2. Sharonda found a pair of white shorts that fit her perfectly. When she noticed they did not have pockets for her tennis balls, though, she put them back on the rack.

Practice: _____

_____ 3. Abdul told the salesperson he needed new workout clothes that were made of natural fibers that would absorb his body perspiration.

Practice: _____

_____ 4. Kenita usually preferred jogging clothes with a loose fit, but she couldn't resist the bright yellow jogging set. Even though it was a little more snug than she liked, the tag read "Reduced 50%." This was just too good to pass up!

Practice: _____

_____ 5. Donovan was excited when his mom gave him money for his birthday. He decided to buy a new set of golf clubs. The local sporting goods store had sold out of the style he preferred, so he settled for a similar style instead. He did not want to wait for the store to reorder his favorite clubs.

Practice: _____

_____ 6. Gerald decided to spend the $100 he had saved for a home gym. He bought a jump rope, a floor mat, and a variety of hand weights.

Practice: _____

_____ 7. Jan had trouble disciplining herself to work out each day. She decided to invest in a year's membership in a nearby gym. There she could work out six days a week with a class of 12 other people.

Practice: _____

_____ 8. Lorraine considered purchasing an exercise bike to put in her apartment. She read consumer articles about the leading models available and studied features in three nearby stores. Lorraine also talked with several friends who had recently bought exercise bikes.

Practice: _____

_____ 9. Mark hurriedly unpacked his new rowing machine. He threw the instruction booklet aside and started rowing.

Practice: _____

(Continued)

_____ 10. Before he decided which pieces of exercise equipment to buy, Eli measured the space he had. He did a scale drawing of the equipment in his room to check for fit.

Practice: _____

_____ 11. Maureen saw the weight loss massage belt advertised on television and immediately called the 800 number to order.

Practice: _____

_____ 12. Jennifer's friends raved about a new workout DVD. Before deciding whether to order the DVD, Jennifer went by the library to check out a copy and preview it.

Practice: _____

_____ 13. Harold's coach advised him to hire a personal trainer to help him prepare for the upcoming weightlifting competition. Harold called the number he saw advertised on the gym bulletin board. He met the trainer, liked him, and hired him on the spot.

Practice: _____

_____ 14. Cecil found a health club that had just the right set of services to suit his exercise needs. The only problem was the club was 40 minutes from his workplace and 50 minutes from his home. He decided to go ahead and join anyway, thinking somehow he would manage it.

Practice: _____

_____ 15. Amy did a cost comparison of the YWCA, a nearby spa, and a community fitness center. This helped her select the best facility to meet her needs.

Practice: _____

_____ 16. John bought a pair of running shoes from a local sports store. Within a week, the inner sole cushions were falling apart. John was very unhappy with the shoes, but he figured that's what happens when you buy inexpensive shoes.

Practice: _____

_____ 17. Austin attempted to get a refund for a defective air pump he had purchased to inflate a raft. The store refused to refund his money, even though he had his receipt. When Austin contacted the manufacturer, he was told the store should return his money. Austin was unsatisfied, so he contacted a government agency about the problem.

Practice: _____

_____ 18. Natalie bought a treadmill for running at home. After she got it home, the treadmill did not work properly. Natalie contacted the store where she had made the purchase. Because she had kept her receipt, the store could easily exchange the treadmill.

Practice: _____

_____ 19. Lucas purchased some boxing gloves for a class he was taking. The week before the first meeting, the class was canceled due to low enrollment. Lucas took his gloves back to the store and demanded a full refund. He did not have a receipt.

Practice: _____

_____ 20. Monica purchased a month's membership at a gym. When she joined, Monica was unaware the gym's showering facilities were unsafe. Her membership was nonrefundable, so Monica decided there was nothing she could do.

Practice: _____

Backtrack
Through Chapter 22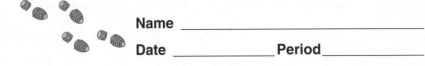

Activity F

Chapter 22

Name _____

Date _____ Period _____

Provide complete answers to the following questions and statements about food and fitness consumer choices.

Recall the Facts

- -

1. What is a consumer? _____

   _____

2. List three advantages food processing offers consumers. _____

   _____

   _____

3. Give two examples of how food processing can affect the chemical and physical characteristics of food products.

   _____

   _____

   _____

4. To which government agency do manufacturers go to seek approval for the use of food additives?

   _____

5. Does research support the belief that organic produce is more nutritious than nonorganic? _____

6. Where should you look to find unit price information in the grocery store? _____

   _____

7. What two agencies regulate food labeling, and what is the area of responsibility of each? _____

   _____

   _____

8. What food products are exempt from labeling laws? _____

   _____

   _____

9. How must ingredients be listed on a label? _____

10. Why do consumers use ingredient lists on labels? _____

    _____

    _____

11. What two basic items are required for taking part in physical activity? _____

    _____

(Continued)

12. What are your rights as a consumer when buying products? _____

_____

Interpret Implications

13. Which three types of food stores do you think are most popular? For each, give two reasons to support your answer.

_____

_____

_____

_____

14. Give one example explaining why an advertiser might want to use persuasive advertising and one example explaining why an advertiser might want to use informational advertising.

_____

_____

15. If organic foods cost more than nonorganic foods, why might a person choose to buy them?

_____

_____

16. Explain why the intended use of a food product affects your choice of national brands, store brands, or generic products. _____

_____

17. Explain the difference between the *sell by* date and the *use by* date on food products. _____

_____

18. Name three parties to whom you may need to issue a complaint as a consumer. _____

_____

Apply & Practice

19. Describe how consumers can use the Nutrition Facts panel on a food product label. _____

_____

_____

20. Review the shopping pointers for fitness products and services found in this chapter. Select the one that would be the most helpful to you and explain how you could implement it. _____

_____

_____